The Complete Hospice Visit

The Complete Hospice Visit

A Nurse's Guide to Excellence

Peter M. Abraham, BSN, RN

The Complete Hospice Visit
A Nurse's Guide to Excellence
Copyright © 2024 Peter M. Abraham, BSN, RN

All rights reserved. No part of this book may be reproduced or transmitted in any manner whatsoever without written permission, except for brief quotations embodied in critical articles and reviews. This book is a work of nonfiction intended for educational purposes only.

This book is a work of non-fiction. The views expressed are solely those of the author and do not necessarily reflect the publisher's opinions, and the publisher disclaims any responsibility for them as a result.

Contact Info: author@2abraham.com

DEDICATION

This book is dedicated to all my fellow hospice nurses; yes, to you! You are out there every workday caring, like me, for the terminally ill – those living in their darkest hours; and here you are bringing light into their day. Thank you!

Table of Contents

Introduction _____ *1*

Chapter 1: An Outline of The Complete Hospice Visit _____ *4*

    The Complete Hospice Visit: A Systematic Approach _____ 4

Chapter 2: Assessing Imminent Death _____ *7*

    Understanding the Two-Week Window _____ 8

    Key Physical Indicators _____ 11

    Communication Protocols _____ 14

    Family Education and Support _____ 16

    Documentation Requirements _____ 18

    Legal Considerations _____ 20

    Conclusion to Chapter 2: Assessing Imminent Death _____ 21

Chapter 3: Evaluating Changes in Condition _____ *22*

    Types of Condition Changes _____ 23

    Assessment Techniques _____ 26

    PRN Visit Planning _____ 29

    Team Communication Strategies _____ 31

    Documentation Best Practices _____ 33

    Conclusion to Chapter 3: Evaluating Changes in Condition _____ 36

Chapter 4: Measuring Decline Velocity _____ *37*

    Understanding Disease Progression _____ 37

Using Assessment Tools 40

Understanding Prognosis Evaluation in Hospice Care 43

Communication with Team and Family 45

Documentation Requirements 47

Conclusion to Chapter 4: Measuring Decline Velocity 49

Chapter 5: Care Plan Effectiveness _____ 50

Elements of an Effective Care Plan 50

Quality of Life Indicators 56

Plan Modification Strategies 58

Documentation Requirements 60

Conclusion to Chapter 5: Care Plan Effectiveness 62

Chapter 6: Medication Management _____ 63

Medication Assessment Protocol 64

Planning for Refills 67

Family Education 69

Coordination with Pharmacy 71

Documentation Requirements 73

Conclusion to Chapter 6: Medication Management 75

Chapter 7: Maximizing Support Services _____ 76

Holistic Assessment in Hospice Care: A Comprehensive Approach 76

Available Support Services 80

Family Resource Assessment 82

Team Coordination 85

Documentation Requirements 87

Conclusion to Chapter 7: Maximizing Support Services 89

Conclusion: Achieving Excellence in Hospice Care _____ 90

Key Takeaways 90

Implementation Strategies 90

Quality Metrics and Outcomes 90

Call to Action for Excellence 91

Continuing Education Resources 91

Appendix A: Assessment Checklists _____ 92

Initial Visit Assessment Checklist 92

Routine Visit Checklist 93

Change in Condition Checklist 93

End-of-Life Checklist 94

Quality Assurance Checklist 94

Appendix B: Documentation Templates _____ 95

Initial Visit Documentation Template 95

Routine Visit Template 96

Change in Condition Template 96

End-of-Life Documentation Template 97

Quality Documentation Elements 98

Appendix C: Communication Scripts _____ 99

Initial Visit Introduction _____ 99

Discussing Changes in Condition _____ 99

Crisis Prevention _____ 100

Family Education _____ 100

Difficult Conversations _____ 100

Support Service Introduction _____ 101

Phone Communication _____ 101

Appendix D: Quick Reference Guides _____ 102

Common Symptom Management _____ 102

Medication Conversion Guide _____ 102

Vital Sign Parameters _____ 102

Emergency Kit Guidelines _____ 103

DME Quick Guide _____ 103

Visit Frequency Guidelines _____ 103

Documentation Essentials _____ 104

Communication Chain _____ 104

Medicare Requirements _____ 104

References and Resources _____ 105

Author Bio _____ 109

Introduction

Achieving Excellence in Hospice Care

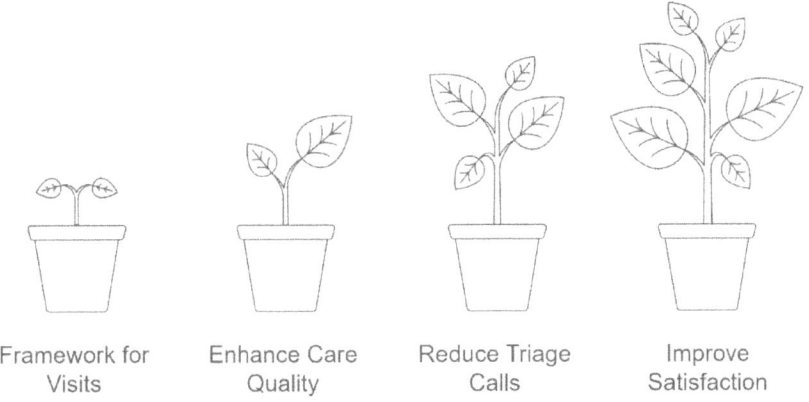

Framework for Visits | Enhance Care Quality | Reduce Triage Calls | Improve Satisfaction

Welcome to "The Complete Hospice Visit: A Nurse's Guide to Excellence." This book is designed to be your trusted companion in providing exceptional end-of-life care. As hospice nurses, we are privileged and responsible for supporting patients and their families during one of life's most challenging journeys. This guide aims to enhance your skills, boost your confidence, and ultimately improve the quality of care you provide.

Purpose and Goals of the Book

The primary purpose of this book is to:

1. Provide a comprehensive framework for conducting thorough hospice visits
2. Enhance the quality of care delivered to patients and their families
3. Reduce unnecessary calls to triage
4. Improve CAHPS scores and overall family satisfaction

Our goals are to:

- Empower you with knowledge and practical skills

- Standardize the assessment process across hospice visits
- Promote proactive care management
- Foster better communication within the hospice team and with families

How to Use This Guide

This book is designed to be both a learning tool and a quick reference guide. Here's how to make the most of it:

1. **Read through each chapter thoroughly:** Read the entire book to understand the assessment process comprehensively. Each chapter will address a component of what needs to be a part of each hospice visit. The first chapter provides an outline with a deeper dive in the chapters that follow.
2. **Practice the techniques:** Apply the assessment strategies daily, refining your skills over time.
3. **Use the checklists:** Refer to the assessment checklists provided in each chapter during your visits.
4. **Refer back as needed:** Keep this guide handy for quick reference when encountering challenging situations.
5. **Share with your team:** Discuss the concepts with your colleagues to promote consistent, high-quality care across your organization.

The Impact of Structured Assessment on Quality of Care

A structured assessment approach can significantly improve the quality of hospice care. Here's how:

Aspect of Care	Impact of Structured Assessment
Patient Comfort	Ensures comprehensive symptom management.
Family Satisfaction	Promotes clear communication and expectation-setting.
Team Efficiency	Facilitates better coordination and resource allocation.
Documentation	Improves accuracy and completeness of patient records.
Care Planning	Enables more targeted and effective interventions.

By implementing a structured assessment process, you can:

- **Identify issues early:** Catch potential problems before they escalate, reducing patient discomfort and family anxiety.
- **Provide consistent care:** Ensure that all aspects of patient care are addressed consistently across all visits.
- **Improve communication:** Facilitate clearer communication within the care team and with the patient's family.
- **Enhance decision-making:** Make more informed decisions about care plans and interventions based on comprehensive assessments.
- **Boost confidence:** Feel more assured in providing high-quality care in various situations.

Remember, structured assessment is not about rigid protocols but ensuring that we consistently provide comprehensive, compassionate care to every patient. As you progress through this book, you'll discover how to blend the art of nursing with the science of structured assessment, ultimately elevating the quality of care you provide to your hospice patients and their families.

In the following chapters, we'll delve into specific aspects of the hospice visit, providing you with the tools and knowledge to excel as a hospice nurse. Let's embark on this journey together, committed to providing excellence in end-of-life care.

Chapter 1: An Outline of The Complete Hospice Visit

The following outlines what a complete hospice visit would look like to improve the quality of care provided, reduce calls to triage, improve CAHPS scores, and overall family satisfaction.

The Complete Hospice Visit: A Systematic Approach

Pre-Visit Preparation

1. Start the visit in the EMR system, including mileage documentation
2. Review the current care plan and recent updates
3. Check previous visit notes for follow-up items

Initial Contact and Assessment

1. Professional introductions as needed
2. Explore the caregiver's observations since the last visit:
   - Changes in condition
   - New or ongoing concerns
   - Effectiveness of interventions

Comprehensive Patient Assessment

1. Patient Interview (when appropriate):
   - Current comfort level
   - Changes in symptoms
   - Concerns or needs
2. Clinical Assessment:
   - Vital signs as appropriate
   - Breathing patterns and effort
   - Functional status
   - Symptom management effectiveness
   - Medication side effects
   - Current prognosis based on caregiver observations, reports, and comprehensive patient assessment

3. Documentation Tools:
    - Update appropriate scales (FAST, KPS, PPS, and others as applicable)
    - Pain assessments (PAINAD if applicable)
    - Nutritional status (MUAC)
    - Other assessments as necessary

Care Delivery and Education

1. Provide necessary treatments:
    - Demonstrate techniques to caregivers
    - Ensure comfort during procedures
    - Validate caregiver understanding
2. Resource Management Review:
    - Medication inventory and expiration dates
    - Supply needs
    - DME functionality and appropriateness

Coordination of Care

1. Contact necessary providers:
    - Pharmacy for refills
    - DME for equipment needs
    - Team members for updates
    - Medical director as needed
2. Plan Ahead:
    - Consider upcoming holidays
    - Account for weather concerns
    - Evaluate the need for PRN visits

Visit Conclusion

1. Education and Updates:
    - Review assessment findings
    - Discuss expected changes
    - Confirm the following visit timing
    - Update care instructions
2. Communication:
    - Contact medical power of attorney if absent
    - Update family members as appropriate
    - Ensure emergency contacts are current

Post-Visit Actions

1. Documentation:
   - Complete visit note
   - Update care plan as needed
   - Record any new orders
2. Team Communication:
   - Update case manager
   - Notify appropriate team members
   - Schedule any needed follow-up

Remember that this systematic approach helps ensure comprehensive care delivery while preventing oversight of critical components during the visit.

Chapter 2: Assessing Imminent Death

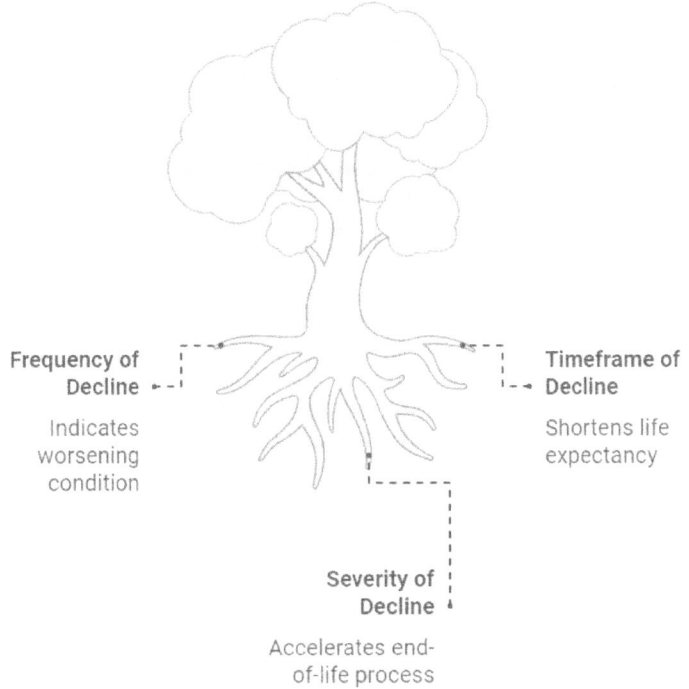

Assessing for imminent death within a two-week window is a critical skill that directly impacts the quality of care provided to hospice patients and their families. This assessment requires keenly observing subtle changes, understanding disease progression patterns, and recognizing when death is approaching. Early recognition of these changes allows the hospice team to adjust care plans proactively, prepare families for what lies ahead, and ensure optimal comfort for the patient.

The ability to identify and respond to signs of imminent death helps prevent crises, reduces unnecessary hospitalizations, and allows families precious time to prepare emotionally and practically. This chapter explores the essential components of this assessment process, including understanding the two-week window, recognizing key physical indicators, implementing effective communication protocols, providing family education and support, and maintaining proper documentation.

The skills involved are mastered over time. Try to keep track of the times you are on target, and when you miss, ask yourself if it were something everyone would have missed or if you could learn from the experience. By mastering these skills, hospice nurses can significantly improve patient care outcomes, family satisfaction, and team coordination during one of life's most significant transitions.

Understanding the Two-Week Window

As I grew as a hospice nurse, I tried not to be hard on myself for missing when I didn't catch the patient in their two-week or less window. However, I encouraged myself to learn from each miss by debriefing and asking what observable signs and symptoms were present that I did not see to learn from the experience. I encourage you to do the same.

The two-week window represents a critical period when changes in a patient's condition accelerate, signaling the approach of death. Understanding the two-week window is one of the most crucial skills you'll develop as a hospice nurse. This period marks a significant transition in the patient's journey, where changes begin to accelerate, signaling the approach to death. Let's explore how to recognize and respond to these changes effectively. It allows you to provide appropriate care and prepare families for what lies ahead.

You'll notice subtle but significant changes early in this window. Patients typically show decreased appetite and fluid intake, transitioning from regular meals to just "bites and sips." Sleep patterns change, with patients spending increasingly more extended periods of sleep. Many begin withdrawing socially and are less interested in previously enjoyed activities or conversations.

Progressive Changes in Breathing

One of the most reliable indicators involves breathing pattern changes. Early in the two-week window, you may notice:

- Irregular breathing rhythms
- Periods of shallow breathing followed by deeper breaths
- Occasional brief pauses in breathing (less than 10 seconds)
- Slight variations from baseline respiratory rate

These breathing changes are distinctly different from late signs like "goldfish breathing" or "fish out of water breathing," which indicate death within hours, not weeks.

Additional Physical Changes

Temperature changes often begin with cool extremities, particularly in the hands and feet. You may notice subtle changes in skin color, especially around the lips or nail beds. These changes typically progress over days, with mottling appearing later.

Behavioral and Consciousness Changes

Patients may experience increased confusion and longer non-responsive periods. Some begin speaking to deceased loved ones or picking at things that aren't present. When patients tell their families they will die soon, take this seriously - they often have an innate awareness of their approaching death.

Assessment Strategy

Focus your assessments on progressive changes, noting:

- Changes in vital signs
- Alterations in consciousness
- Decreasing oral intake
- Temperature fluctuations
- Skin color changes

Remember that these changes build upon each other, creating a comprehensive picture of decline. Your role is to recognize these patterns early, allowing you to prepare families and adjust care plans appropriately. Each patient's journey through this window may vary, but understanding these patterns enables timely, appropriate care interventions.

Velocity of Changes

Frequency of Change	Typically Means Death Within
One every 4-8 weeks	Less than 6 months
Every 3-4 weeks	Less than 3 months
Every 1-2 weeks	Less than 2 months
Once every week	Less than 1 month
Several times per week	Less than 2 weeks
Every day	Less than 1 week
Several times per day	Less than 72 hours

Key Trigger Words and Observations

Physical Changes

- "Goldfish breathing" or "fish out of water breathing" (late sign)
- "Taking guppy breaths" (late sign)
- "Sleeping more than awake"
- "Eating bites and sips"
- Cool extremities (late sign)
- Mottling of skin (middle to late sign)

Behavioral Changes

- Increased confusion
- Non-responsive periods
- Speaking to deceased loved ones
- Picking at things not present
- Telling family they will die soon
- Increased weakness

Assessment Focus Points

Early Signs

- Decreased appetite and fluid intake
- Increased sleep periods
- Social withdrawal
- Changes in vital signs
- Skin color changes

Progressive Signs

- Significant decline in oral intake
- Pronounced breathing changes
- Altered consciousness
- Temperature fluctuations
- Further withdrawal

Late Signs

- Minimal to no oral intake
- Cheyne-Stokes breathing
- Mottling of extremities
- Decreased urine output
- Decreased consciousness

Understanding these changes within the two-week window helps nurses anticipate needs, adjust care plans appropriately, and prepare families for the changes they will observe. Each patient's journey through this window may vary, but recognizing these patterns enables timely, appropriate care interventions.

Key Physical Indicators

When assessing for the two-week window of imminent death, it's crucial to recognize early indicators that signal the beginning of this period. When observed collectively, these signs help determine the progression toward the end of life and allow for timely interventions and family preparation.

Respiratory Changes

Early Breathing Pattern Changes

- Irregular breathing rhythms
- Periods of shallow breathing followed by deeper breaths
- Occasional brief pauses in breathing (less than 10 seconds)
- Slight increase or decrease in respiratory rate from baseline

Progression to Watch For

- More frequent and noticeable pauses in breathing
- "Fish out of water" or "guppy" breathing (mouth opening and closing)
- Increased use of accessory muscles
- Audible congestion or "rattling" in the chest

Circulatory Changes

Early Skin Signs

- Slight coolness in extremities, particularly hands and feet
- Subtle changes in skin color, especially around the lips or nail beds
- Slower capillary refill

Progression to Monitor

- Increasing coolness spreading up extremities
- Paleness or grayish tone to the skin
- Early signs of mottling, typically starting on knees, feet, or hands

Neurological Changes

Initial Consciousness Changes

- Increased periods of sleep
- Difficulty maintaining focus or attention
- Subtle changes in the ability to communicate

Progression to Observe

- Longer periods of unresponsiveness
- Difficulty rousing from sleep
- Changes in ability to swallow safely

Elimination Changes

Early Output Indicators

- Gradual decrease in urinary output
- Changes in urine color or concentration
- Decreased frequency of bowel movements

Progression to Note

- Significant reduction in urinary output
- Very concentrated or dark urine
- Constipation or reduced bowel sounds

Functional Decline

Initial Changes

- Increased weakness
- Reduced ability to perform ADLs independently
- Spending more time in bed or recliner

Progression to Watch For

- Inability to get out of bed
- Difficulty changing positions without assistance
- Reduced muscle tone

System	Early Indicators	Progression to Monitor
Respiratory	Irregular rhythms, slight changes in rate	"Fish out of water" breathing, increased pauses
Circulatory	Slight coolness in extremities, subtle color changes	Increasing coolness, early mottling

System	Early Indicators	Progression to Monitor
Neurological	Increased sleep, difficulty focusing	Longer unresponsive periods, swallowing changes
Elimination	Gradual decrease in output, color changes	Significant reduction in output, very concentrated urine
Functional	Increased weakness, reduced ADL ability	Bed-bound, difficulty changing positions

Assessment Tips

- **Observe Trends:** Look for patterns of change over time rather than isolated observations.
- **Document Progression:** Note how quickly changes are occurring.
- **Use Family Input:** Family members often notice subtle changes first.
- **Consider Baseline:** Compare current status to the patient's typical condition.
- **Holistic Approach:** Consider all systems together for a comprehensive assessment.

Remember, when assessed together and in the context of the patient's overall condition, these physical indicators provide valuable insight into the progression of the dying process. Early recognition of these signs allows for proactive care planning and timely support for the patient and their family.

Communication Protocols

Effective communication during the two-week window is crucial for coordinating care, supporting families, and ensuring optimal patient comfort. Clear, timely, and compassionate communication helps prevent crises and improves outcomes for all involved.

Team Communication

Priority Updates to Report

- Changes in vital signs, especially breathing patterns
- New symptoms or concerns
- Medication effectiveness

- Family dynamics or needs
- Changes in functional status
- Nutritional intake changes
- New safety concerns

Communication Timing

Urgency Level	When to Communicate	To Whom
Immediate	Active symptoms, safety issues	Case Manager, On-Call Nurse
Within 2 Hours	New concerning changes	Primary Care Team
Within 24 Hours	Routine updates, stable changes	IDT Members
Next Visit	General observations, stable status	Next Visiting Nurse

Documentation Essentials

Key Elements to Record

- Objective findings
- Subjective observations
- Family teaching provided
- Response to interventions
- Updates to the care plan
- Follow-up needed

Family Communication Guidelines

Essential Topics to Address

- Current status changes
- Expected progression
- Medication adjustments
- Comfort measures
- When to call hospice
- Available support services

Communication Techniques

Best Practices

- Use clear, non-medical language
- Validate family observations
- Provide written instructions
- Confirm understanding
- Document conversations
- Set expectations for next steps

Remember that effective communication during this period helps prevent unnecessary hospitalizations, reduces families' anxiety, and ensures continuity of care across the hospice team.

Family Education and Support

Key Educational Topics

Physical Changes to Explain

- Decreased appetite and thirst
- Changes in sleeping patterns
- Breathing pattern changes
- Temperature fluctuations
- Skin color changes
- Reduced awareness of surroundings

Comfort Measures to Teach

- Proper positioning techniques
- Mouth care methods
- Skin care approaches
- Safe feeding practices
- Managing restlessness
- Creating a peaceful environment

Supporting Family Needs

Emotional Support

- Acknowledge feelings and fears
- Validate their observations
- Listen to their concerns
- Respect cultural beliefs
- Support spiritual needs
- Encourage self-care

Practical Support

- Review the medication schedule and remaining supply
- Demonstrate care techniques
- Explain equipment use
- Discuss respite options
- Review emergency plans
- Share resource information

Teaching Methods

Approach	Best Used For	Examples
Demonstration	Hands-on care	Positioning, mouth care
Written materials	Complex information	Medication schedules
Verbal instruction	Simple concepts	When to call hospice
Return demonstration	Skill verification	Safe transfers

Signs Requiring Contact

Teach Families to Call When

- New or worsening symptoms
- Changes in breathing patterns
- Increased restlessness
- Pain control issues
- Medication questions

- Emotional distress
- Safety concerns

Family Preparedness

Help Families Plan For

- Medication refills
- Equipment needs
- Visitor management
- Final arrangements
- Emergency situations
- Support system activation

Remember that well-educated and supported families provide better patient care and experience less anxiety during this challenging time. Regular reinforcement of teaching points helps ensure understanding and compliance with the care plan.

Documentation Requirements

Proper documentation during the two-week window is crucial for ensuring continuity of care, meeting regulatory requirements, and supporting the best possible patient outcomes. Accurate and comprehensive documentation also facilitates effective communication among team members and provides a legal record of care provided. Please consider buying the ***Compliance-based, Eligibility Driven Hospice Documentation: Tips for Hospice Nurses*** book on Amazon for a deeper dive into audit-proofing your documentation and helping you keep eligible patients on service.

Essential Elements to Document

Patient Status

- Vital signs and trends (only if not already handled in the EMR)
- Physical assessment findings
- Changes in condition
- Symptom presence and severity
- Functional status changes
- Nutritional intake
- Elimination patterns

Interventions and Responses

- Medications administered
- Non-pharmacological interventions
- Patient's response to treatments
- Effectiveness of comfort measures
- Equipment use and functionality

Family Interactions

- Education provided
- Family's understanding of information
- Emotional state of family members
- Support services offered or requested
- Family's ability to provide care

Care Planning

- Updates to the plan of care
- Goals of care discussions
- Advance directive reviews
- Interdisciplinary team recommendations

Documentation Best Practices

1. **Be Objective:** Use factual observations rather than subjective interpretations.
2. **Be Specific:** Include measurable data and precise descriptions.
3. **Be Timely:** Document as soon as possible after observations or interventions.
4. **Be Comprehensive:** Include all relevant information, even if it seems minor.
5. **Be Accurate:** Double-check all entries for correctness.
6. **Be Legible:** Ensure all handwritten notes are clear and readable.

Documentation Frequency

Situation	Minimum Documentation Frequency
Routine visit	Every visit
Symptom changes	As they occur
Medication changes	Immediately upon change
Family education	Each teaching session
Care plan updates	At least weekly

Key Phrases for Documentation

- "Patient appears to be actively dying as evidenced by..."
- "Family educated on signs of imminent death, including..."
- "Comfort measures implemented with the following results..."
- "Plan of care updated to address..."
- "Family verbalizes understanding of..."
- "Last visit _____ compared to this visit _____"

Avoiding Common Documentation Pitfalls

- **Don't** use vague terms like "appears comfortable" without supporting evidence.
- **Don't** include personal opinions or non-professional observations.
- **Don't** use abbreviations that your organization does not approve.
- **Don't** leave blank spaces or lines in your documentation.
- **Don't** alter previous documentation without following proper procedures.

Legal Considerations

- Document all phone calls, including time, content, and response.
- Note any refusals of care or treatment, including the reason given.
- Record any unusual incidents or accidents promptly and thoroughly.
- Include family members present during visits or discussions.
- Document any concerns about safety or potential abuse/neglect.

Remember, thorough and accurate documentation ensures quality patient care and protects you and your organization legally. It's a critical component of professional nursing practice, especially during this sensitive time in the patient's care.

Conclusion to Chapter 2: Assessing Imminent Death

Accurate assessment of imminent death within the two-week window represents one of the most critical skills a hospice nurse can develop. By carefully observing and documenting changes in physical indicators, maintaining clear communication with the team and family, providing comprehensive education and support, and maintaining thorough documentation, you create an environment where patients can experience a peaceful death while families feel supported and prepared.

Remember that each patient's journey is unique, and your expertise in recognizing these patterns allows for proactive rather than reactive care. When you successfully identify the two-week window, you give families the precious gift of time - time to gather, say goodbye, complete essential tasks, and begin their grief journey with support and understanding.

Your role in this assessment process directly impacts the quality of care provided and how families will remember their hospice experience. By implementing the practices outlined in this chapter, you help fulfill hospice's promise of providing excellent end-of-life care while supporting families through one of life's most challenging transitions.

Chapter 3: Evaluating Changes in Condition

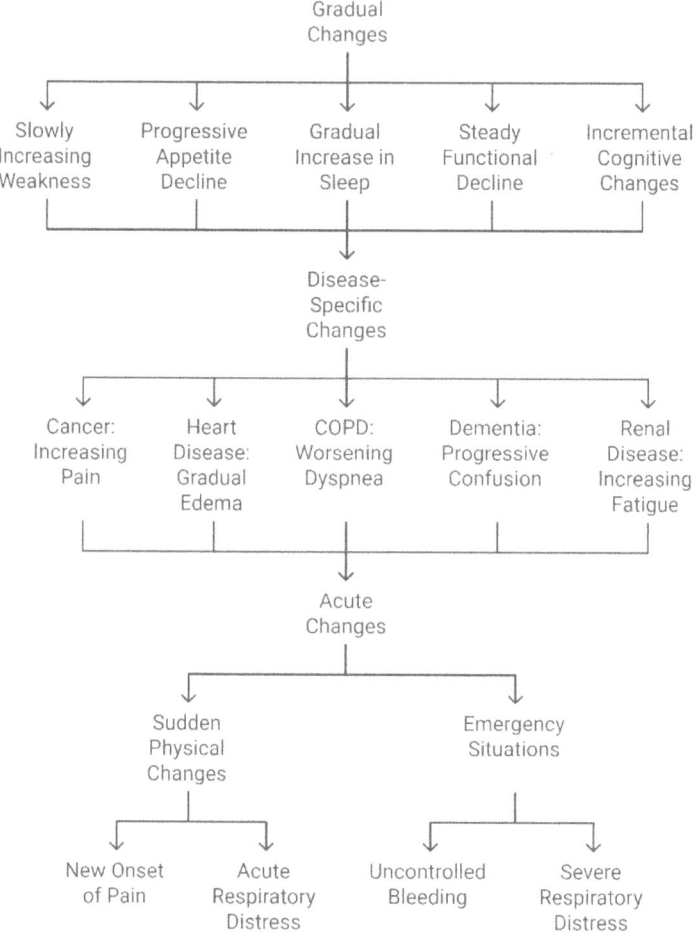

Evaluating changes in a hospice patient's condition requires keen observation, systematic assessment, and clear communication. The ability to recognize and respond appropriately to these changes directly impacts patient comfort, family satisfaction, and quality of care. Whether the changes are gradual or sudden, expected or unexpected, your skilled evaluation determines the appropriate interventions and support needed.

This chapter explores the various types of condition changes you may encounter, provides structured assessment techniques, guides PRN visit planning, outlines effective team communication strategies, and details documentation best practices. By mastering these essential skills, you'll be better equipped to provide proactive rather than reactive care, ultimately improving patient and family outcomes.

Types of Condition Changes

Understanding the various types of condition changes helps hospice nurses differentiate between expected disease progression and acute changes requiring immediate intervention. These changes generally fall into several categories requiring different approaches and responses.

Expected Disease Progression

When caring for hospice patients, you'll observe two main expected changes: gradual and disease-specific. Gradual changes typically follow a predictable pattern, with patients showing slowly increasing weakness, progressive appetite decline, and incremental cognitive changes. These changes often occur over weeks to months and represent the natural progression of terminal illness.

Disease-specific changes vary based on the underlying diagnosis. For instance, cancer patients commonly experience increasing pain and tumor growth, while heart disease patients show gradual increases in edema. COPD patients typically demonstrate slowly worsening dyspnea. Understanding these patterns helps you anticipate and proactively address emerging needs.

Gradual Changes

- Slowly increasing weakness
- Progressive appetite decline
- Gradual increase in sleep
- Steady functional decline
- Incremental cognitive changes

Disease-Specific Changes

- Cancer: Increasing pain, tumor growth
- Heart Disease: Gradual increase in edema

- COPD: Slowly worsening dyspnea
- Dementia: Progressive confusion
- Renal Disease: Increasing fatigue

Acute Changes

Acute changes require immediate attention and often signal a significant shift in the patient's condition. They can manifest as a new onset of pain, acute respiratory distress, sudden confusion, or rapid functional decline. When observed, these changes often indicate a need for immediate intervention and care plan modification.

Sudden Physical Changes

- New onset of pain
- Acute respiratory distress
- Sudden confusion
- Falls or injuries
- Rapid decline in function

Emergency Situations

- Uncontrolled bleeding
- Severe respiratory distress
- New fractures
- Acute neurological changes
- Unrelieved pain

Velocity of Change

The speed at which changes occur provides valuable prognostic information. When changes happen gradually over months, this typically indicates a longer prognosis. However, when multiple changes occur within days or weeks, this often signals the approaching end of life. For example, if a patient shows rapid changes in functionality, mental status, and vital signs within a short period, this typically indicates a shorter prognosis.

Speed of Change	Timeframe	Example
Gradual	Weeks to months	Slowly decreasing appetite

Speed of Change	Timeframe	Example
Moderate	Days to weeks	Increasing weakness
Rapid	Hours to days	Acute pain crisis
Immediate	Minutes to hours	Respiratory distress

Psychosocial Changes

Remember that decline isn't purely physical. Watch for behavioral changes such as increased anxiety, new depression, or social withdrawal. These changes often precede or accompany physical decline and require equal attention. Family dynamic changes, including new caregiver stress or family conflicts, can significantly impact care delivery and require prompt intervention.

Behavioral Changes

- Increased anxiety
- New Depression
- Social withdrawal
- Personality changes
- Sleep pattern disruption

Family Dynamic Changes

- New caregiver stress
- Family conflicts
- Support system changes
- Financial concerns
- Grief reactions

Environmental Changes

Changes in the patient's environment can dramatically affect their care needs. Pay attention to safety concerns, equipment needs, and changes in caregiver availability. These factors often determine whether the current care plan remains appropriate or needs modification.

Home Situation

- Safety concerns
- Equipment needs
- Caregiver availability
- Living arrangement changes
- Access to resources

Understanding these different types of changes helps determine the following:

- Urgency of response needed
- Type of intervention required
- Level of family support needed
- Communication Priorities
- Documentation requirements

Remember that changes rarely occur in isolation. A change in one area typically triggers or reflects changes in others. For example, physical decline often leads to increased caregiver stress, which may then affect the patient's emotional state. This interconnected nature of changes requires you to maintain a comprehensive assessment approach, considering all aspects of the patient's condition and circumstances.

Understanding these various changes and their implications allows you to anticipate needs better, adjust care plans appropriately, and support patients and families through the hospice journey.

Assessment Techniques

Effective assessment of condition changes requires a systematic approach, combining keen observation with targeted questioning and physical examination. The following techniques will help you gather comprehensive information to guide clinical decision-making.

Systematic Physical Assessment

Head-to-Toe Approach

1. Neurological: Level of consciousness, orientation, speech
2. Respiratory: Rate, depth, pattern, use of accessory muscles
3. Cardiovascular: Pulse, blood pressure, skin color/temperature
4. Gastrointestinal: Bowel sounds, distension, output
5. Genitourinary: Urine output, color, odor
6. Musculoskeletal: Strength, mobility, edema
7. Skin: Color, temperature, integrity, wounds

OLDCARTS Method for New Symptoms

- Onset: When did it start?
- Location: Where is it?
- Duration: How long does it last?
- Characteristics: What does it feel like?
- Aggravating factors: What makes it worse?
- Relieving factors: What makes it better?
- Timing: Is there a pattern?
- Severity: Rate on a scale of 0-10

Observation Techniques

Non-Verbal Cues

- Facial expressions
- Body posture
- Restlessness or stillness
- Interaction with environment
- Response to stimuli

Environmental Clues

- Medication organization
- Home cleanliness
- Presence of adaptive equipment
- Safety hazards
- Family interactions

Targeted Questioning

Open-Ended Questions

- "Tell me about any changes you've noticed."
- "How has your typical day changed recently?"
- "What concerns you most right now?"

Focused Questions

- "Have you had any new pain since my last visit?"
- "How many times did you use the bathroom today?"
- "Are you able to walk to the bathroom independently?"

Functional Assessment

Activity	Independent	Needs Assistance	Dependent
Bathing			
Dressing			
Toileting			
Transferring			
Feeding			

Pain Assessment

Comprehensive Pain Evaluation

- Location
- Intensity (0-10 scale)
- Quality (sharp, dull, aching, etc.)
- Radiation
- Timing (constant, intermittent)
- Exacerbating/alleviating factors

Cognitive Assessment

Quick Cognitive Screen

- Orientation to person, place, time
- Short-term memory (recall 3 words after 5 minutes)
- Simple calculation (100-7 serially)
- Clock drawing test

Family/Caregiver Input

Key Questions for Caregivers

- "What changes have you noticed?"
- "How are you managing with care?"
- "What's been most challenging for you?"
- "Do you have any concerns about medications?"

Remember, effective assessment combines objective data with subjective information from the patient and family. Your clinical judgment, informed by these comprehensive assessment techniques, guides the care plan and ensures timely interventions.

PRN Visit Planning

Planning for PRN (as needed) visits requires careful consideration of patient needs, symptom management, and regulatory requirements. Effective PRN visit planning helps prevent crises and ensures continuity of care.

During your current visit, you should ask yourself if you need to plan for a PRN visit either later the same day or within what time frame. These pre-planned PRN visits help improve outcomes and ensure the patient and family members that your focus is on the patient.

PRN Visit Requirements

Essential Components of PRN Orders

- Specific description of symptoms that trigger a visit
- Clear parameters for intervention

- Defined number of visits allowed
- Time frame for the visits
- Documentation requirements

Qualifying PRN Visits

Component	Required Elements	Example
Symptoms	Specific triggers	Pain rated > 6/10
Frequency	Defined limit	1-2x/week
Duration	Time period	For 2 weeks
Parameters	Clear indicators	For new onset SOB
Follow-up	Next steps	Reassess in 24 hours

Planning Considerations

Assessment Factors

- Recent changes in condition
- Pattern of symptom occurrence
- Family/caregiver capabilities
- Available support systems
- Distance to patient's home

Implementation Strategies

- Schedule follow-up within 24 hours of condition changes
- Plan visits during times of known symptom exacerbation
- Coordinate with other disciplines as needed
- Consider front-loading visits during periods of instability

Documentation Elements

Required Information

- Date and time of visit
- Reason for PRN visit

- Assessment findings
- Interventions provided
- Response to interventions
- Plan for follow-up
- Communication with team members

Remember that PRN visits are vital for managing changing conditions and preventing hospitalizations. Proper planning and documentation ensure regulatory compliance and optimal patient care.

As a rule of thumb, if the patient's condition changes, the patient was placed on a new medication (especially an opioid, benzodiazepine, or related medication that may require careful monitoring for dose effectiveness and side effects), or your nursing gut tells you, plan for a PRN visit the next day or so.

Team Communication Strategies

Effective team communication is crucial for providing high-quality hospice care. By implementing robust communication strategies, hospice nurses can ensure seamless coordination, improve patient outcomes, and enhance family satisfaction.

Interdisciplinary Team Meetings

Regular interdisciplinary team meetings are essential for coordinating care and sharing important patient information. These meetings should:

- Be held weekly to discuss patient care, symptom management, and emotional support needs
- Include all relevant team members, such as nurses, physicians, social workers, and chaplains
- Provide an opportunity for open dialogue and collaborative problem-solving
- Allow for updates on patient condition, care plan adjustments, and family concerns

Utilizing Technology for Communication

Leveraging technology can significantly enhance team communication:

- **Electronic Health Records (EHRs):** Ensure all team members have access to up-to-date patient information
- **Secure Messaging Platforms:** Enable quick and efficient communication among team members
- **Telehealth Tools:** Facilitate remote consultations and decision-making

Clear Role Delineation and Leadership

Establishing clear roles and leadership within the team improves communication:

- Designate a liaison staff member as a point of contact for coordinating team efforts
- Clearly define each team member's responsibilities to prevent confusion or duplication of efforts
- Encourage open communication across all levels of the team hierarchy

Promoting Trust and Collaboration

Building strong relationships within the team fosters better communication:

- Create an atmosphere where all team members feel comfortable expressing opinions and asking questions
- Encourage interdisciplinary collaboration to leverage diverse expertise
- Regularly acknowledge and appreciate team members' contributions

Communication Documentation

Proper documentation ensures continuity of care and clear communication:

Documentation Element	Purpose
Visit notes	Record patient status, interventions, and responses
Care plan updates	Track changes in treatment approach
Team meeting minutes	Summarize discussions and decisions made
Family communication logs	Document interactions with the patient's family

Strategies for Effective Communication

1. **Active Listening:** Focus entirely on the speaker, understand their message, and respond appropriately
2. **Clear and Concise Language:** Avoid medical jargon when communicating with patients and families
3. **Empathy:** Acknowledge the feelings and concerns of patients, families, and team members
4. **Cultural Sensitivity:** Respect diverse backgrounds and adapt communication styles accordingly
5. **Regular Check-ins:** Schedule brief daily huddles to address immediate concerns and updates

By implementing these communication strategies, hospice nurses can foster a collaborative environment that enhances patient care, supports team cohesion, and ultimately improves the quality of hospice services provided

Documentation Best Practices

Clear, accurate documentation supports quality patient care, ensures regulatory compliance, and facilitates effective team communication when evaluating changes in condition.

Essential Documentation Elements

Change in Condition Documentation

- Specific symptoms or changes observed
- Time and date of onset
- Severity and frequency
- Impact on daily activities
- Interventions attempted
- Response to interventions
- Follow-up plan

SBAR Format for Documentation

Component	Content	Example
Situation	A brief statement of the current status	"Patient experiencing increased SOB"
Background	Relevant history and context	"History of COPD with recent decline"
Assessment	Clinical findings and analysis	"Respiratory rate 28, using accessory muscles"
Recommendation	Plan and next steps	"Implemented oxygen protocol, scheduling follow-up"

Objective vs. Subjective Documentation

Objective Findings

- Vital signs with trends
- Physical assessment findings
- Observable symptoms
- Measurable changes
- Equipment readings

Subjective Information

- Patient complaints
- Family concerns
- Reported symptoms
- Comfort levels
- Emotional status

Documentation Timing

Critical Elements

- Document changes immediately
- Record interventions as performed
- Note communication with team members
- Track medication administration
- Update care plan changes

Quality Assurance Elements

Documentation Must Be

- Clear and concise
- Accurate and complete
- Timely and relevant
- Legible and organized
- Professional in tone

Remember that thorough documentation supports continuity of care, meets regulatory requirements, provides legal protection, and ensures optimal patient outcomes.

Conclusion to Chapter 3: Evaluating Changes in Condition

Evaluating changes in condition represents a cornerstone of excellent hospice nursing care. Your ability to recognize, assess, and respond to these changes ensures that patients receive timely interventions and appropriate support. Through systematic assessment, thoughtful PRN visit planning, effective team communication, and thorough documentation, you create a comprehensive care approach that anticipates and addresses patient needs before they become crises.

Remember that each change you observe, document, and communicate about contributes to the larger picture of patient care. Your expertise in evaluating these changes improves patient comfort and family satisfaction, strengthens team collaboration, and ensures regulatory compliance. Implementing the strategies outlined in this chapter helps create a caring environment where changes are met with confidence, competence, and compassion.

Chapter 4: Measuring Decline Velocity

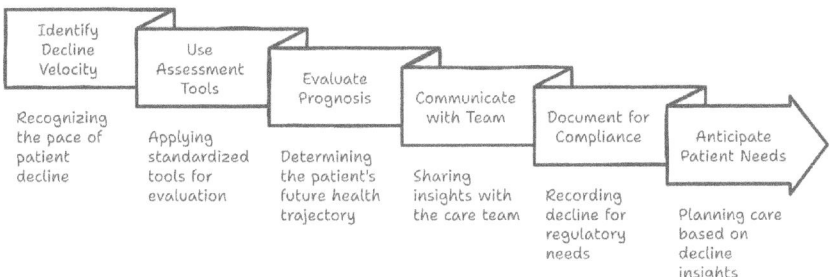

Measuring decline velocity is a critical skill for hospice nurses. It provides valuable insights into a patient's disease progression and guides care decisions. This chapter explores the nuances of understanding and documenting the pace of decline, which directly impacts care planning, resource allocation, and family preparation.

We'll delve into the patterns of disease progression across various conditions, examine the use of standardized assessment tools, and discuss strategies for evaluating prognosis. Additionally, we'll cover effective communication techniques for sharing this information with the care team and families, ensuring everyone is aligned in understanding the patient's journey.

Proper documentation of decline velocity is essential for regulatory compliance and continuity of care. Mastering these skills will better equip you to anticipate patient needs, provide proactive care, and support families through the hospice experience.

Understanding Disease Progression

Understanding disease trajectories is essential for providing proactive, patient-centered hospice care. Let's explore how different disease patterns progress and what this means for your clinical practice.

Disease Trajectory Patterns

These are only a sampling of disease projection patterns.

Cancer Trajectory: The Rapid Decline Pattern

Cancer patients typically maintain relatively good function until near the end of life. When decline begins, it often progresses rapidly over weeks to days. For example, a patient with advanced lung cancer might be independently managing daily activities and then experience a sharp, functional decline marked by increased weakness, decreased appetite, and escalating pain.

Cancer patients typically maintain relatively good function until near the end of life. When decline begins, it often progresses rapidly over weeks to days. For example, a patient with advanced lung cancer might be independently managing daily activities and then experience a sharp functional decline marked by increased weakness, decreased appetite, and escalating pain. This pattern requires you to:

- Prepare families for sudden changes
- Plan for rapid escalation of services
- Ensure comfort medications are in place before urgent need
- Schedule more frequent visits during the decline phase

Organ Failure Trajectory: The Roller Coaster

Patients with conditions like heart failure or COPD follow what's often called a "stair-step" or "roller coaster" pattern. They experience episodes of acute deterioration followed by partial recovery, though never quite returning to their previous baseline. This unpredictable pattern means you should:

- Educate families about the pattern of good and bad days
- Develop clear crisis management plans
- Adjust visit frequency based on current status
- Focus on preventing avoidable exacerbations

Frailty/Dementia Trajectory: The Long Decline

The frailty trajectory, common in dementia and general debility, shows the slowest progression. These patients experience gradual functional loss over months to years. This extended trajectory requires:

- Long-term caregiver support strategies
- Regular reassessment of care needs
- Prevention of complications

- Close monitoring for subtle changes

Understanding these trajectories helps predict care needs and guide resource allocation. For instance, cancer patients typically need intensive services for a shorter period, while dementia patients require sustained lower-intensity support over a longer time.

While these patterns are typical, individual patients may not follow them strictly. Your ongoing assessment and clinical judgment remain crucial in providing appropriate care.

Measuring Velocity of Decline

Timeframe of Changes	Velocity Level	Clinical Significance
Monthly	Gradual	Expected disease progression
Weekly	Moderate	Approaching end-stage
Daily	Rapid	Likely terminal phase
Hourly	Precipitous	Imminent death likely

Key Indicators of Progression

Physical Indicators

- Changes in vital signs
- Functional decline
- Symptom progression
- Nutritional status
- Energy levels

Functional Indicators

- Activities of Daily Living (ADLs)
- Mobility changes
- Sleep patterns
- Social engagement
- Cognitive function

Understanding disease progression helps predict care needs, guide resource allocation, and prepare families for changes. This knowledge forms the foundation for effective hospice care planning and delivery.

Using Assessment Tools

Assessment tools provide the foundation for measuring and documenting decline velocity in hospice patients. Understanding how to select and implement these tools effectively helps ensure accurate tracking of patient progression while supporting clinical decision-making.

The book *Mastering Hospice Eligibility: An Essential Guide for RNs and Clinical Managers* covers a broader range of assessment tools and includes instructions for their use.

The Palliative Performance Scale (PPS) is one of our primary assessment tools, measuring functional status across multiple domains. When using the PPS, evaluate the patient's ambulation, activity level, self-care ability, oral intake, and level of consciousness. For example, a patient who declines from PPS 60% to 40% over two weeks demonstrates a significant change that may indicate approaching end-of-life.

The Edmonton Symptom Assessment System (ESAS) is another crucial measurement tool. It uses a 0-10 scale to evaluate nine key symptoms. When implementing ESAS, remember that it captures the patient's subjective experience of symptoms like pain, tiredness, and shortness of breath. Using ESAS regularly helps track symptom progression and evaluate treatment effectiveness.

Consistency is key to the effective implementation of these tools. Use the same assessment tool at each visit to establish clear trends. Rather than focusing on isolated scores, look for patterns of change over time. For instance, if a patient's ESAS scores for fatigue and drowsiness steadily increase over several visits, this may indicate disease progression.

When documenting your findings, focus on trends and changes rather than just numbers. Include these changes' impact on care planning and note the patient's and family's response to declining scores. This comprehensive approach helps the entire team understand what is changing and how these changes affect the patient's overall care needs.

Remember that while these tools provide valuable objective data, they should support rather than replace your clinical judgment. Use them as part of your comprehensive patient evaluation, combining the scores with your observations, patient and family input, and clinical expertise to guide care decisions.

By mastering these assessment tools, you'll be better equipped to track decline velocity accurately and adjust care plans proactively, ultimately providing better support for your patients and their families through the end-of-life journey.

Primary Assessment Tools

Palliative Performance Scale (PPS)

- Measures functional status
- Tracks changes in condition
- Evaluates:
    - Ambulation
    - Activity level
    - Self-care ability
    - Oral intake
    - Level of consciousness

Edmonton Symptom Assessment System (ESAS)

- Uses 0-10 scale for key symptoms:
    - Pain
    - Tiredness
    - Nausea
    - Depression
    - Anxiety
    - Drowsiness
    - Appetite
    - Well-being
    - Shortness of breath

Specialized Assessment Tools

Tool	Purpose	Best Used For
FAST Scale	Dementia progression	Alzheimer's/dementia patients
AKPS	Activity and self-care ability	General functional assessment
PCPSS	Problem severity screening	Overall symptom burden
RUG-ADL	Motor function assessment	Activities of daily living

Implementation Guidelines

For Effective Tool Use:

- Select appropriate tools based on diagnosis
- Use consistently across visits
- Document trends rather than isolated scores
- Share findings with team members
- Adjust care plan based on results

Documentation Requirements

Essential Elements to Record:

- Tool scores at each visit
- Changes from previous assessments
- Impact on care planning
- Patient/family response
- Team communication needs

Remember that assessment tools support clinical judgment but should not replace it. Use them as part of a comprehensive evaluation of the patient's condition and decline velocity.

Understanding Prognosis Evaluation in Hospice Care

Evaluating prognosis in hospice care requires both clinical expertise and careful observation. Let's explore how to effectively combine assessment tools with decline patterns to make informed prognostic decisions.

When evaluating physical indicators, pay close attention to how frequently changes occur. A patient showing weekly changes typically has a shorter prognosis than one with monthly changes. For example, suppose you notice vital signs becoming unstable, nutritional intake declining rapidly, and consciousness levels fluctuating within the same week. In that case, this pattern suggests a shorter prognosis than gradual changes over months.

Disease-specific markers provide valuable prognostic information. Watch for signs like increasing oxygen requirements or declining kidney function in organ failure. With cancer patients, observe tumor progression through symptoms like increasing pain or new metastatic sites. The rate of change in these markers often indicates prognosis more accurately than any single measurement.

Functional assessment correlation, particularly using the PPS (Palliative Performance Scale), helps quantify decline. A patient whose PPS score drops from 60% to 40% in two weeks typically has a shorter prognosis than one who maintains a stable 50% for several months. When scores fall into the 30-40% range, this often indicates a prognosis of weeks to months, while scores of 10-20% suggest days to weeks.

Documentation plays a crucial role in prognosis evaluation. Beyond recording changes, document the pattern and velocity of decline. Include both objective findings and clinical observations. For example, note that the patient is sleeping more and quantify the increase in sleep hours and associated functional impacts.

Remember that prognosis evaluation isn't just about predicting timing - it guides resource allocation and helps prepare families. When you identify a changing prognosis, use this information to adjust visit frequency, modify care plans, and initiate essential family discussions about what to expect.

By systematically combining these elements, you can develop more accurate prognostic evaluations that support clinical decision-making and family preparation.

Key Prognostic Indicators

Physical Indicators

- Frequency of condition changes
- Velocity of functional decline
- Changes in vital signs
- Nutritional status
- Level of consciousness

Disease-Specific Markers

- Organ failure progression
- Tumor growth or spread
- Infection frequency
- Wound healing capacity
- Response to treatments

Decline Patterns and Prognosis

Frequency of Changes	Typical Prognosis	Required Actions
Every 3-4 months	6 months or less	Regular monitoring
Monthly	2-3 months	Increase visit frequency
Weekly	Weeks to 1 month	Update care plan
Daily	Days to weeks	Prepare for end-of-life
Multiple times daily	Hours to days	Initiate imminent death care

Functional Assessment Correlation

PPS Score Correlation

- 70-100%: Extended prognosis
- 50-60%: Months
- 30-40%: Weeks to months
- 10-20%: Days to weeks

Documentation Elements

Essential Components

- Changes in condition
- Decline patterns
- Tool scores
- Clinical observations
- Family understanding

Remember that prognosis evaluation guides resource allocation, family preparation, and care planning while helping maintain appropriate hospice eligibility documentation.

Communication with Team and Family

Effective communication about decline velocity is crucial for coordinating care and preparing families for changes. Clear, compassionate communication ensures everyone involved understands the patient's progression and can make informed decisions.

Team Communication

Key Information to Share

- Changes in assessment scores
- New symptoms or concerns
- Alterations in care needs
- Family dynamics or concerns
- Recommendations for care plan adjustments

Communication Methods

1. Daily team huddles
2. Weekly IDT meetings
3. Secure messaging platforms
4. EHR updates
5. Shift change reports

Family Communication

Essential Discussion Points

- Current status and recent changes
- Expected progression
- Potential upcoming needs
- Available support services
- Decision-making considerations

Communication Strategies

- Use clear, non-medical language
- Provide written summaries
- Encourage questions
- Validate emotions and concerns
- Offer ongoing support

Timing of Communications

Decline Velocity	Team Communication	Family Communication
Gradual	Weekly updates	Monthly family meetings
Moderate	Bi-weekly updates	Bi-weekly family check-ins
Rapid	Daily updates	Frequent family discussions
Precipitous	Continuous updates	Daily family meetings

Addressing Difficult Topics

Strategies for Sensitive Discussions

- Choose the appropriate setting
- Allow ample time
- Use empathetic language
- Provide emotional support
- Offer follow-up resources

Remember that clear, consistent communication about decline velocity helps prevent crises, reduces family anxiety, and ensures the entire care team is aligned in providing appropriate support.

Documentation Requirements

Accurate documentation of decline velocity provides essential clinical information, supports Medicare eligibility, and ensures continuity of care. Proper documentation helps demonstrate the appropriateness of hospice care and guides care planning decisions.

Core Documentation Elements

Every Visit Documentation

- Current PPS/FAST scores
- Changes from previous visit
- New symptoms or concerns
- Functional status changes
- Response to interventions
- Family understanding

Decline Velocity Indicators

- Frequency of changes
- Pattern of decline
- Impact on daily activities
- Changes in care needs
- Support system adjustments

Required Timeframes

Documentation Type	When to Complete	Purpose
Visit Notes	Within 24 hours	Record current status
Change Reports	Immediately	Alert team to changes
Weekly Summaries	Every 7 days	Track progression
Recertification	Every 60/90 days	Support Eligibility

Medicare Requirements

Essential Components

- Observable decline patterns
- Objective measurements
- Disease progression evidence
- Functional status changes
- Terminal prognosis support

Supporting Documentation

- Assessment tool scores
- Physical findings
- Symptom progression
- Care plan updates
- Team communications

Quality Assurance Elements

Documentation Must Be

- Clear and objective
- Timely and accurate
- Comprehensive
- Professionally written
- Properly authenticated

Remember that thorough documentation meets regulatory requirements and supports quality patient care and effective team communication.

Conclusion to Chapter 4: Measuring Decline Velocity

Measuring decline velocity is an essential skill that empowers hospice nurses to provide proactive, compassionate care. By understanding disease progression, utilizing assessment tools effectively, and evaluating prognosis accurately, you can anticipate and address patient needs with precision and empathy.

Clear communication about decline velocity with your team and the patient's family ensures everyone is aligned in their understanding and expectations. This shared knowledge fosters trust, reduces anxiety, and allows for more informed decision-making.

Remember, thorough documentation of decline velocity meets regulatory requirements, supports continuity of care, and demonstrates the ongoing need for hospice services. Your expertise in measuring and documenting decline velocity directly contributes to improved patient comfort, family satisfaction, and overall quality of care.

As you apply these skills in your daily practice, you'll find yourself better equipped to navigate the complexities of end-of-life care, providing invaluable support to patients and families during one of life's most challenging journeys.

Chapter 5: Care Plan Effectiveness

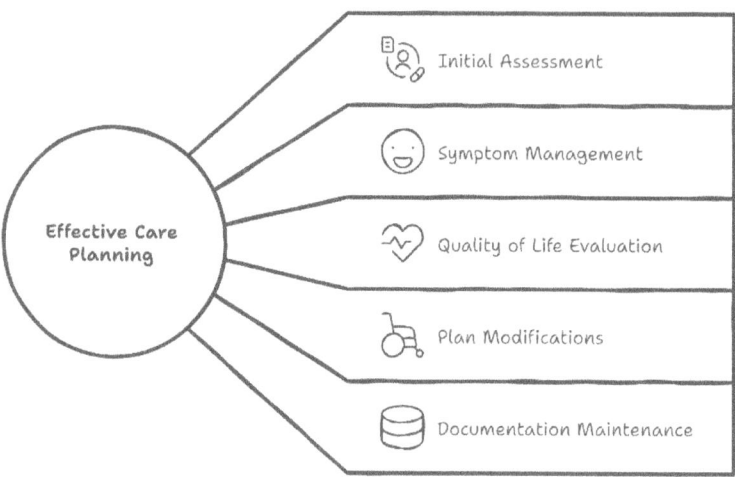

Creating and maintaining effective care plans lies at the heart of quality hospice care. A well-crafted care plan is both a roadmap for delivering comprehensive patient care and a communication tool for the entire hospice team. When properly developed and implemented, it ensures that all aspects of patient care are addressed while meeting regulatory requirements.

This chapter explores the essential elements of effective care planning, from initial assessment through ongoing modifications. We'll examine how to conduct thorough symptom management assessments, evaluate quality of life indicators, implement strategic plan modifications, and maintain proper documentation. Understanding these components helps ensure that care remains patient-centered, responsive to changing needs, and focused on optimal outcomes.

By mastering these aspects of care planning, you'll be better equipped to provide comprehensive, coordinated care that enhances patient comfort and family satisfaction while meeting regulatory requirements.

Elements of an Effective Care Plan

A well-crafted hospice care plan is a roadmap for delivering comprehensive, patient-centered care. Understanding and implementing these essential elements ensures optimal outcomes and regulatory compliance. The book

Care Plans for Hospice Patients: A Comprehensive Guide dives deeper into hospice care plans.

Core Components

Patient-Specific Goals

- Symptom management targets
- Comfort measures
- Quality of life objectives
- Functional status goals
- Psychosocial needs

Problem Identification

- Current symptoms
- Potential complications
- Risk factors
- Family concerns
- Support needs

Interventions and Approaches

Problem Area	Interventions	Expected Outcomes
Pain	Medication protocol, positioning	Comfort achieved
Respiratory	Breathing techniques, oxygen	Easier breathing
Anxiety	Medications, counseling	Reduced distress
ADLs	Support services, equipment	Maintained dignity
Family Support	Education, resources	Enhanced coping

Required Elements

Medicare Requirements

- Measurable goals
- Specific interventions

- Timeframes for review
- Discipline responsibilities
- Outcome measures

Safety Considerations

- Fall Prevention
- Medication management
- Emergency protocols
- Equipment needs
- Environmental safety

Individualization Factors

Patient-Specific Elements

- Cultural preferences
- Spiritual needs
- Family dynamics
- Living situation
- Support system

Care Coordination

- IDT involvement
- Family participation
- Community resources
- Volunteer services
- Spiritual care

Remember that an effective care plan is dynamic, requiring regular review and updates to reflect changing patient needs and circumstances. It serves as a clinical guide and a communication tool for the entire hospice team. Symptom Management Assessment

Effective symptom management is a cornerstone of quality hospice care. A comprehensive assessment ensures patients receive timely, appropriate interventions to maximize comfort and quality of life.

Key Symptoms to Assess

1. **Pain**
   - Location
   - Intensity (0-10 scale)
   - Quality (sharp, dull, aching)
   - Timing (constant, intermittent)
   - Aggravating/alleviating factors
2. **Respiratory Distress**
   - Dyspnea severity
   - Oxygen saturation
   - Use of accessory muscles
   - Presence of cough or secretions
3. **Gastrointestinal Issues**
   - Nausea/vomiting
   - Constipation/diarrhea
   - Appetite changes
   - Abdominal discomfort
4. **Neurological Symptoms**
   - Level of consciousness
   - Confusion/delirium
   - Seizure activity
   - Weakness/paralysis
5. **Psychological Distress**
   - Anxiety
   - Depression
   - Agitation
   - Insomnia

Assessment Tools

Tool	Purpose	When to Use
ESAS	Overall symptom burden	Every visit.
PAINAD	Pain in non-verbal patients	Every visit is a good way to contrast the patient's report with objective visual observations.

Tool	Purpose	When to Use
CAM	Delirium screening	With mental status changes.
HADS	Anxiety and depression	Weekly (the Hospital Anxiety and Depression Scale is considered a reliable and valid tool for screening anxiety and depression in palliative care patients.

Your hospice team may use scales/tools other than those mentioned above. The key is to use those scales every visit consistently.

Comprehensive Symptom Assessment: A Practical Guide

Understanding how to conduct thorough symptom assessments is fundamental to providing excellent hospice care. Let's explore how to effectively use the OPQRSTUV method to gather comprehensive information about patient symptoms.

Using OPQRSTUV Effectively

When a patient or caregiver reports a symptom, systematically work through each component of OPQRSTUV to build a complete picture. For example, if a patient reports pain:

Start with **Onset**: "When did this pain begin? Was it sudden or gradual?" This helps establish a timeline and potential causes.

Move to **Provoking/Palliating** factors: "What makes the pain worse? What brings relief?" These answers guide intervention choices and help patients maintain comfort.

Explore **Quality**: Ask patients to describe the sensation in their own words. Different descriptors (sharp, burning, aching) often indicate different underlying causes and guide treatment approaches.

For **Region/Radiation**, have patients point to where they feel the symptom and trace any movement or spread. This information helps track disease progression and determine appropriate interventions.

When assessing **Severity**, use consistent scales (0-10) and ask about the best and worst times. This provides baseline data for tracking intervention effectiveness.

Timing patterns help predict and prevent symptom exacerbations: "Does it come and go? Is it worse at certain times?"

Understanding the patient's perspective about the cause often reveals fears or misconceptions that need addressing.

Values assessment helps prioritize interventions based on what matters most to the patient.

Evaluating Intervention Effectiveness

After implementing interventions, systematic reassessment is crucial. Document baseline severity before intervention, then track changes using the same assessment method. This consistency helps identify trends and determine if adjustments are needed.

Regular caregiver input provides valuable perspective on symptom management effectiveness between visits. Their observations often reveal patterns or concerns that patients might not express directly.

Remember that comprehensive assessment isn't just about gathering data - it's about understanding the full impact of symptoms on both patient and family to guide effective care planning.

OPQRSTUV Method

- Onset: When did it start?
- Provoking/Palliating: What makes it better or worse?
- Quality: What does it feel like?
- Region/Radiation: Where is it? Does it spread?
- Severity: How intense is it (0-10)?
- Timing: Is it constant or intermittent?
- Understanding: What does the patient think is causing it?
- Values: How is this impacting quality of life?

Intervention Effectiveness Evaluation

For Each Symptom:

- Document baseline severity
- Record interventions used
- Assess response to treatment
- Note any side effects
- Determine the need for plan adjustments

Family/Caregiver Input

Key Questions:

- "What changes have you noticed?"
- "How effective do you think the current treatments are?"
- "Are there any new concerns since our last visit?"
- "How is managing symptoms affecting you?"

Remember, thorough symptom assessment forms the foundation for effective care planning and intervention. Regular reassessment ensures the care plan remains responsive to the patient's changing needs.

Quality of Life Indicators

Quality of life assessment forms a crucial component of effective hospice care planning. Understanding and monitoring these indicators helps ensure that care remains focused on patient comfort and satisfaction.

Core Quality Domains

Physical Comfort

- Pain management effectiveness
- Symptom control
- Physical comfort level
- Sleep Quality
- Energy levels

Emotional Well-being

- Psychological comfort
- Anxiety levels
- Depression screening
- Emotional support
- Sense of peace

Social Connections

- Family relationships
- Social engagement
- Communication ability
- Visitor interactions
- Support system involvement

Measurement Components

Domain	Indicators	Assessment Method
Physical	Symptom control	Symptom scales
Psychological	Emotional state	Mood assessment
Social	Family dynamics	Observation/interview
Spiritual	Religious needs	Spiritual assessment
Functional	Independence level	ADL assessment

Patient-Centered Indicators

Daily Living Quality

- Preferred location of care
- Maintenance of independence
- Achievement of personal goals
- Dignity preservation
- Comfort with care team

Support System Assessment

- Family involvement
- Caregiver well-being
- Resource utilization
- Support service effectiveness
- Communication satisfaction

Quality Measurement Tips

Assessment Strategies

- Use patient self-reporting when possible
- Include caregiver observations
- Document trends over time
- Note the impact of interventions
- Track satisfaction levels

Remember that quality of life is highly individual and subjective. Regular assessment helps ensure care plans align with patient preferences and goals while maintaining optimal comfort and dignity.

Plan Modification Strategies

Care plan modifications ensure hospice care remains responsive to changing patient needs and circumstances. A systematic approach to plan modification helps maintain quality care while meeting regulatory requirements.

Triggers for Plan Modification

Clinical Changes

- New or worsening symptoms
- Changes in functional status
- Altered medication needs
- Equipment requirements
- Safety concerns

Psychosocial Changes

- Family coping difficulties

- Changes in support system
- New emotional needs
- Spiritual care needs
- Environmental changes

Implementation Process

Required Steps

- Review current goals and outcomes
- Assess the effectiveness of interventions
- Document changes in condition
- Update care strategies
- Communicate with team members

Timing of Updates

Situation	Update Required	Documentation Needed
Routine Review	Every 15 days	Care plan review notes
Condition Changes	Immediately	Comprehensive assessment
Level of Care Change	Within 24 hours	Updated goals and interventions
New Symptoms	As they occur	Modified interventions

Quality Assurance Elements

Essential Components

- Measurable outcomes
- Specific interventions
- Clear timeframes
- Team responsibilities
- Patient/family input

Collaborative Approach

Team Integration

- Include all disciplines
- Obtain family input
- Consider patient preferences
- Incorporate caregiver feedback
- Update all team members

Remember that care plan modifications should reflect the patient's changing needs and the family's ability to provide care. Regular assessment and timely updates ensure continuous quality care delivery.

Documentation Requirements

Proper documentation of care plan effectiveness ensures regulatory compliance, supports quality care delivery, and facilitates team communication. Clear, comprehensive documentation demonstrates the ongoing need for hospice services while tracking patient outcomes.

Essential Documentation Elements

Care Plan Reviews

- Current status evaluation
- Progress toward goals
- Effectiveness of interventions
- Changes in condition
- Updates to plan of care

Required Timeframes

Documentation Type	Frequency	Purpose
Initial Care Plan	Within 5 days	Establish baseline
Comprehensive Assessment	Every 15 days	Track progress
IDT Reviews	Every 15 days	Team coordination

Documentation Type	Frequency	Purpose
Plan Updates	As needed	Address changes

Outcome Measurements

Key Areas to Document

- Symptom management effectiveness
- Functional status changes
- Quality of life indicators
- Family/caregiver coping
- Support service utilization

Progress Notes Requirements

- Objective findings
- Subjective observations
- Intervention responses
- Family education provided
- Follow-up needed

Medicare Compliance Elements

Required Components

- Terminal prognosis support
- Skilled care necessity
- Service intensity justification
- Goal progression
- Level of care appropriateness

Quality Assurance Documentation

Focus Areas

- Care plan problems
- Interventions provided
- Expected outcomes
- Actual outcomes
- Plan modifications

Remember that thorough documentation meets regulatory requirements, supports continuity of care, and demonstrates the value of hospice services.

Conclusion to Chapter 5: Care Plan Effectiveness

Effective care planning serves as the foundation for delivering exceptional hospice care. By incorporating comprehensive symptom management, monitoring the quality of life indicators, and implementing timely plan modifications, you create a dynamic framework that responds to each patient's unique needs and circumstances.

Remember that a care plan is more than just a document—it's a living tool that guides the entire team in providing coordinated, compassionate care. Through careful assessment, regular updates, and thorough documentation, you ensure that care remains focused on patient comfort and family support while meeting regulatory requirements.

Your expertise in developing and maintaining effective care plans directly impacts patient outcomes, family satisfaction, and team coordination. As you apply these principles in your daily practice, you contribute to the highest standard of hospice care delivery, honoring both your professional commitment and the sacred trust placed in you by patients and families.

Chapter 6: Medication Management

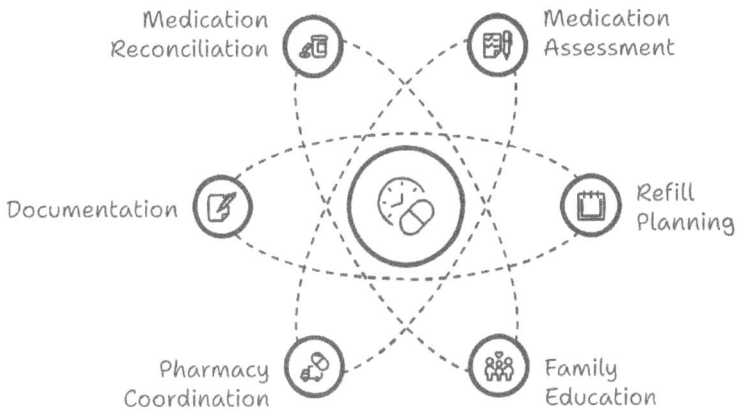

Medication management is critical to hospice care, directly impacting patient comfort and quality of life. As a hospice nurse, your expertise in this area ensures patients receive optimal symptom relief while minimizing risks associated with medication use.

This chapter explores the key aspects of effective medication management in hospice care. We'll delve into comprehensive medication assessment protocols, strategies for proactive refill planning, essential family education techniques, effective coordination with pharmacy services, and crucial documentation requirements.

While this chapter deals with the every-visit component of medication management, anytime there is a change in the patient's condition, or at least quarterly, there should be a deeper dive into medication reconciliation, looking at what medications should be deprescribed or started; the book *Medication Reconciliation in Hospice Care: Maximizing Quality of Life* covers these topics in depth.

By mastering these elements, you'll be better equipped to provide safe, effective medication management that enhances patient comfort, supports family caregivers, and meets regulatory standards. Your skills in this area are vital to preventing medication-related problems, ensuring continuous symptom control, and ultimately improving the quality of life for patients and their families during this sensitive time.

Medication Assessment Protocol

Effective medication management is one of your most critical responsibilities as a hospice nurse. Let's explore how to conduct thorough medication assessments that ensure patient safety and comfort while supporting family caregivers.

Start each medication assessment with a comprehensive reconciliation. Review the current medication list against what's actually in the home, including all prescriptions, over-the-counter medications, supplements, and herbals. Pay special attention to recently discontinued medications - these often cause confusion for families and may still be present in the home.

When evaluating effectiveness, look beyond simple symptom control. Observe how medications work together, their timing, and any side effects. For example, if pain medications are making a patient too drowsy to interact with family, the dosing schedule might need adjustment even if the pain is well-controlled.

Caregiver competency assessment is crucial. Watch caregivers demonstrate medication administration techniques and listen to their explanation of each medication's purpose. This hands-on observation often reveals issues that aren't apparent through conversation alone. Common problems include confusion about PRN medication timing or uncertainty about when to report side effects.

The comfort kit requires special attention. Beyond checking medication availability and expiration dates, ensure families understand exactly when and how to use each medication. Many caregivers feel anxious about using comfort kit medications - clear education and written instructions help build their confidence.

Watch for red flags that might indicate problems:

- Medication hoarding often signals fear about pain or symptom management
- Confusion about medication regimens may indicate overwhelming caregiver stress
- Missing medications could suggest financial concerns or diversion issues

Remember that medication assessment isn't a one-time task. Regular reassessment helps prevent complications and ensures that symptom management remains effective as the patient's condition changes.

Conducting thorough medication assessments helps ensure safe and effective symptom management while supporting family caregivers in their vital role.

Core Assessment Components

Medication Reconciliation

- Current medication list
- Recently discontinued medications
- Over-the-counter products
- Supplements and herbals
- PRN medication usage patterns

Effectiveness Evaluation

- Symptom control
- Side effect presence
- Dosing adequacy
- Administration timing
- Drug interactions

Safety Assessment

Assessment Area	Key Elements	Action Items
Storage	Temperature, security	Address safety concerns
Organization	Sorting, labeling	Set up medication system
Administration	Proper technique, timing	Provide education
Disposal	Unused medications	Document disposal
Documentation	MAR completion	Ensure accuracy

Caregiver Competency

Essential Skills to Assess

- Medication administration technique
- Understanding of medication purpose
- Recognition of side effects
- Proper documentation
- Emergency protocols

Education Needs

- Medication schedules
- Administration methods
- Storage requirements
- When to call hospice
- Disposal procedures

Comfort Kit Assessment

Key Elements

- Medication availability
- Expiration dates
- Storage conditions
- Usage instructions
- Family understanding

Remember that thorough medication assessment helps prevent complications, ensures effective symptom management, and supports family confidence in providing care.

Red Flag Indicators

Watch For:

- Medication hoarding
- Confusion about regimens
- Inappropriate usage
- Missing medications
- Administration errors

Regular medication assessment ensures safe and effective symptom management while supporting family caregivers in their vital role.

Planning for Refills

Proactive refill planning prevents medication gaps, reduces family stress, and ensures continuous symptom management. A systematic approach to refill planning helps maintain optimal comfort and prevent crises. By staying on top of medication needs, you reduce calls to triage and increase patient and family satisfaction.

Assessment Timeline

Medication Review Schedule

- Every visit: Check current supplies
- Weekly: Project refill needs
- Bi-weekly: Review comfort kit status
- Monthly: Evaluate the overall medication plan

Supply Monitoring

Medication Type	Check When	Action Needed
Routine meds	7-day supply remains	Initiate refill
PRN meds	50% remaining	Assess refill need
Comfort kit (unopened)	Monthly	Replace if expired
Comfort kit (in use)	Every visit	Assess each medication's remaining doses; replace individual medications as needed
Controlled substances	3-day supply remains	Priority refill

Coordination Process

Essential Steps

- Contact pharmacy
- Verify insurance coverage
- Arrange delivery
- Confirm receipt
- Document process

Special Considerations

- After-hours needs
- Weekend coverage
- Holiday planning
- Weather concerns
- Transportation issues

Family Education

Key Teaching Points

- How to monitor supplies
- When to request refills
- Emergency procedures
- Pharmacy contacts
- Documentation needs

Documentation Requirements

Record Keeping

- Current medication list
- Refill requests
- Delivery confirmation
- Family Education
- Follow-up needs

Remember that proactive refill planning prevents medication gaps and reduces stress for both families and the hospice team while ensuring continuous symptom management.

Emergency Planning

Contingency Measures

- Backup pharmacy options
- Emergency kit protocols
- After-hours procedures
- Alternative delivery methods
- Family emergency plans

Effective refill planning supports continuous comfort care while preventing unnecessary anxiety and crises.

Family Education

Educating families about medication management is crucial for patient comfort and safety in hospice care. Effective education empowers caregivers to manage medications while confidently reducing stress and potential errors.

Key Educational Topics

1. Medication Purpose and Benefits

- Explain the role of each medication in symptom management
- Discuss how medications contribute to overall comfort

2. Proper Administration Techniques

- Provide step-by-step instructions for each medication
- Demonstrate correct administration methods
- Address special considerations (e.g., crushing pills, using liquid forms)

3. Recognizing and Managing Side Effects

- Identify common side effects for each medication
- Teach how to monitor for adverse reactions
- Guide when to contact the hospice team

4. Safe Storage and Disposal

- Outline best practices for medication storage
- Explain proper disposal methods for unused medications
- Discuss the importance of keeping medications secure

5. When to Contact Hospice

- List scenarios requiring immediate communication
- Provide clear guidelines for reporting concerns
- Emphasize the 24/7 availability of hospice support

Education Strategies

Strategy	Description	Benefits
Written materials	Provide clear, concise handouts	Reinforces verbal instructions
Teach-back method	Ask caregivers to explain in their own words	Ensures understanding
Hands-on practice	Guide caregivers through medication tasks	Builds confidence
Follow-up calls	Check-in regularly to address questions	Provides ongoing support

Addressing Common Concerns

- **Fear of opioids:** Explain the importance of pain management and address misconceptions
- **Medication interactions:** Discuss potential interactions and how to avoid them
- **Adherence challenges:** Provide tips for creating medication schedules and reminders

Remember that family education is an ongoing process. Regularly assess caregiver understanding and provide additional support to ensure optimal medication management and patient comfort.

Coordination with Pharmacy

Effective coordination with pharmacy services ensures timely medication delivery and optimal symptom management for hospice patients. Building strong relationships with pharmacy partners helps prevent medication delays and supports quality patient care.

Essential Communication Elements

Regular Pharmacy Updates

- Medication changes and discontinuations
- New symptoms requiring intervention
- Changes in patient status
- Emergency medication needs
- Supply monitoring concerns

Clinical Collaboration

- Medication reviews every 15 days
- Participation in care planning
- Drug interaction monitoring
- Alternative medication recommendations
- Deprescribing opportunities

Pharmacy Partnership Components

Area	Responsibilities	Outcomes
Clinical Review	Medication appropriateness, interactions	Enhanced safety
Supply Management	Inventory monitoring, timely refills	Continuous care
Cost Management	Formulary compliance, generic alternatives	Resource optimization
Emergency Support	After-hours access, urgent deliveries	Crisis prevention

Pharmacy Service Models

Key Considerations

- Local pharmacy partnerships
- Mail-order services
- Pharmacy benefit managers (PBM)
- Emergency medication access
- Delivery systems

Quality Assurance Measures

Monitoring Elements

- Medication availability
- Delivery timelines
- Communication effectiveness
- Cost management
- Service Satisfaction

Remember that strong pharmacy partnerships contribute significantly to patient comfort and family satisfaction while helping prevent medication-related problems.

Best Practices

Partnership Enhancement

- Regular communication channels
- Clear roles and responsibilities
- Emergency protocols
- Quality metrics
- Performance reviews

Effective pharmacy coordination ensures medications are available when needed while supporting optimal symptom management and cost-effective care delivery.

Documentation Requirements

Proper medication documentation ensures patient safety, regulatory compliance, and effective communication among team members. Clear, accurate documentation supports quality care delivery while meeting Medicare requirements.

Essential Documentation Elements

Every Visit Documentation

- Current medication list review
- Effectiveness assessment
- Side effect monitoring
- Supply status
- Changes in regimen

Medication Changes

- Reason for change
- New orders received
- Discontinuation details
- Patient/family education
- Response to changes

Required Timeframes

Documentation Type	When Required	Purpose
Medication Profile	Initial and updates	Current medication record
Effectiveness Review	Every visit	Symptom management
Comfort Kit Review	Every visit when in use	Supply management
Medication Changes	Within 24 hours	Care coordination
Education Provided	Same day as teaching	Compliance support

Medicare Requirements

Key Components

- Medical Necessity
- Appropriate interventions
- Response to therapy
- Ongoing need
- Cost-effectiveness

Safety Documentation

Critical Elements

- Storage compliance
- Administration technique
- Caregiver competency
- Disposal records
- Safety concerns

Remember that thorough medication documentation supports patient safety, demonstrates appropriate care, meets regulatory requirements, and facilitates team communication.

Quality Assurance Elements

Documentation Must Be

- Clear and accurate
- Timely and complete
- Objective and specific
- Properly authenticated
- Readily accessible

Effective medication documentation ensures continuity of care while supporting regulatory compliance and quality assurance efforts.

Conclusion to Chapter 6: Medication Management

Effective medication management represents one of the most crucial responsibilities in hospice nursing. Through systematic assessment, proactive refill planning, comprehensive family education, coordinated pharmacy partnerships, and thorough documentation, you create a foundation for optimal symptom management and patient comfort.

Remember that your expertise in medication management directly impacts patient outcomes and family confidence in providing care. By consistently implementing these strategies, you help prevent medication-related problems, ensure continuous symptom control, and support families through their caregiving journey.

Your attention to medication management details - from assessment through documentation - demonstrates professional excellence while fulfilling hospice's promise of comprehensive comfort care. As you apply these principles in your daily practice, you contribute significantly to the quality of life for patients and their families during this important time.

Chapter 7: Maximizing Support Services

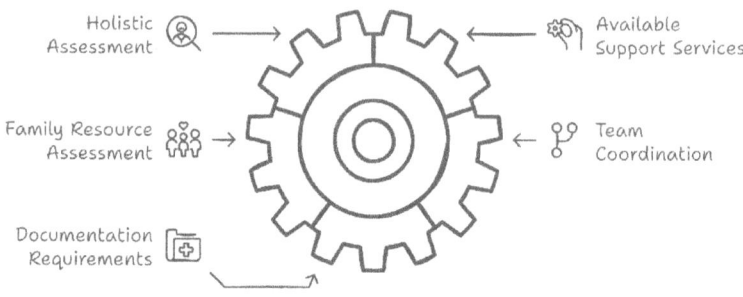

Maximizing support services is essential for providing comprehensive hospice care that truly meets the needs of patients and their families. As a hospice nurse, your ability to identify, coordinate, and implement appropriate support services directly impacts the quality of care and family satisfaction with hospice services.

This chapter explores the key components of effective support service utilization, beginning with a holistic assessment approach that considers all aspects of patient and family needs. We'll examine the range of available support services, discuss strategies for assessing family resources, outline effective team coordination methods, and review essential documentation requirements.

Understanding how to maximize support services helps ensure that patients and families receive the comprehensive care they need while maintaining regulatory compliance and promoting optimal outcomes throughout the hospice journey.

Holistic Assessment in Hospice Care: A Comprehensive Approach

A holistic assessment forms the cornerstone of excellent hospice care, looking beyond physical symptoms to understand the complete picture of a patient's and family's needs. Let's explore how to conduct these assessments effectively in your daily practice.

When conducting a physical domain assessment, evaluate current symptoms and how they impact daily life. For example, when assessing functional limitations, observe how these affect both the patient's independence and the caregiver's ability to provide care. Safety requirements should be evaluated within the context of the home environment - what works in one setting may need modification in another.

The emotional and psychological domain requires particular sensitivity. When assessing coping mechanisms, observe both verbal and non-verbal cues. Are family members showing signs of stress while saying they're managing well? Depression screening should be ongoing, as emotional needs often change as physical decline progresses.

Social domain assessment goes beyond simply listing available support. Consider the strength and sustainability of the support system. For instance, if adult children take turns providing care, evaluate how well this arrangement works and whether it can be maintained as needs increase. Financial resources often directly impact care choices - understanding these constraints early helps develop realistic care plans.

The spiritual domain deserves equal attention, though many nurses feel less comfortable. Remember that spirituality extends beyond religious preferences. Some patients find meaning through nature, music, or family connections. Understanding these sources of support helps integrate them meaningfully into the care plan.

Implementation requires careful coordination. When matching needs with resources, consider timing and sequencing. For example, if a patient needs physical therapy and spiritual support, which should come first? How can services be scheduled to maximize benefits while minimizing family overwhelm?

Remember that holistic assessment is dynamic - what you learn today may change tomorrow. Regular reassessment helps catch changes early and adjust support services accordingly. This proactive approach helps prevent crises and supports better patient and family outcomes.

By conducting thorough holistic assessments, you create a foundation for truly comprehensive hospice care that addresses all aspects of the end-of-life journey.

Core Assessment Domains

Physical Domain

- Symptom management needs
- Functional limitations
- Safety requirements
- Equipment needs
- Personal care assistance

Emotional/Psychological Domain

- Coping mechanisms
- Anxiety levels
- Depression screening
- Grief manifestations
- Family dynamics

Social Domain

- Support system strength
- Financial resources
- Cultural considerations
- Community connections
- Caregiver availability

Spiritual Domain

- Religious preferences
- Faith-based support
- Cultural practices
- End-of-life rituals
- Spiritual distress

Assessment Integration

Domain	Assessment Tools	Support Services
Physical	PPS, ESAS	Nursing, Aide Services
Emotional	HADS, PHQ-9	Social Work, Counseling
Social	Support Assessment	Volunteers, Community Resources
Spiritual	Spiritual Distress Scale	Chaplain, Faith Community

Key Assessment Principles

Comprehensive Evaluation

- Consider all domains equally
- Identify interconnections
- Recognize cultural influences
- Account for family dynamics
- Address barriers to care

Assessment Timing

- Initial evaluation
- Regular reassessment
- Change in condition
- Family request
- Crisis intervention

Remember that holistic assessment forms the foundation for effective support service utilization and optimal patient care outcomes.

Implementation Strategies

Service Coordination

- Match needs with resources
- Consider timing of services
- Integrate team approaches
- Monitor effectiveness

- Adjust support as needed

A thorough holistic assessment ensures that all patient and family needs are identified and addressed through appropriate support services.

Available Support Services

Hospice care offers a comprehensive range of support services designed to address the multifaceted needs of patients and their families. As hospice nurses, our ability to coordinate and maximize support services directly impacts patient care quality and family coping. Let's explore how to assess and implement these vital services effectively.

When evaluating support service needs, start with core medical and nursing services. Beyond providing direct care like pain management and wound care, consider how these services integrate with the family's caregiving routine. For example, when teaching medication administration, schedule training sessions when multiple family members can participate, increasing the support network's capability.

Personal care assistance requires careful coordination. When arranging hospice aide visits, consider the patient's physical needs and the family's schedule and preferences. Some families may need early morning assistance for bathing, while others prefer evening help with bedtime routines.

Emotional and psychological support often requires a gentle introduction. Many families initially decline counseling services but may become more receptive as their needs evolve. Watch for signs of caregiver stress or anticipatory grief that might indicate the need for additional support.

Core Support Services

Medical and Nursing Care

- Pain and symptom management
- Medication administration and monitoring
- Wound care and dressing changes
- Vital sign monitoring

Personal Care Assistance

- Bathing and grooming
- Dressing and toileting
- Mobility assistance
- Light housekeeping

Emotional and Psychological Support

- Counseling services for patients and families
- Support groups
- Anxiety and depression management
- Coping strategies education

Spiritual Care

- Chaplain services
- Spiritual guidance and rituals
- Cultural sensitivity in care planning
- End-of-life spiritual support

Specialized Support Services

Service	Description	Benefits
Respite Care	Short-term inpatient care to relieve caregivers	Prevents caregiver burnout
Therapy Services	Physical, occupational, and speech therapy	Maintains function and comfort
Nutritional Counseling	Dietary advice and meal planning	Supports overall well-being
Music and Art Therapy	Creative expression for emotional processing	Enhances quality of life

Family and Caregiver Support

Education and Training

- Medication management instruction
- Safe patient handling techniques
- Recognizing and reporting changes in condition
- End-of-life care preparation

Practical Assistance

- Help with errands and household tasks
- Coordination of medical equipment and supplies
- Assistance with financial and legal matters
- Connection to community resources

Bereavement Services

- Pre-death counseling for anticipatory grief
- Individual and group grief counseling
- Memorial services and remembrance events
- Resource libraries for grief education

Remember that these support services are designed to work together, providing comprehensive care that addresses all aspects of the patient's and family's needs. Your role as a hospice nurse includes direct care provision and coordinating and facilitating access to these vital support services.

Family Resource Assessment

Understanding family dynamics is crucial for effective service implementation. Start by identifying the primary caregiver and their support network. Observe how decisions are made within the family - is there one clear decision-maker, or does the family operate by consensus? This understanding helps you tailor service recommendations appropriately.

When assessing caregiver capacity, look beyond physical ability. Consider emotional readiness, time constraints, and technical competence. A physically capable caregiver who works full-time may need different support than a retired spouse who's always present but has limited strength.

Pay particular attention to gaps in support. Common challenges include:

- Coverage for overnight care
- Transportation to medical appointments
- Meal preparation and household maintenance
- Respite care for primary caregivers

Remember that resource needs change throughout the hospice journey. Regular reassessment helps identify emerging needs before they become crises. For example, a caregiver who initially manages well may need increased support as the patient's condition declines.

By understanding both available services and family resources, you can create a comprehensive support plan that evolves with changing needs while maintaining family confidence and patient comfort.

Core Assessment Areas

Family Structure and Dynamics

- Primary caregiver identification
- Available family support network
- Family communication patterns
- Decision-making processes
- Cultural considerations

Caregiver Capacity

- Physical ability to provide care
- Emotional readiness
- Time availability
- Technical skills and knowledge
- Need for additional training

Resource Evaluation

Resource Type	Assessment Focus	Support Needed
Physical Support	Home environment, equipment needs	Medical supplies, safety modifications

Resource Type	Assessment Focus	Support Needed
Emotional Support	Coping mechanisms, stress levels	Counseling, support groups
Financial Resources	Available funds, insurance coverage	Financial planning, benefit assistance
Community Support	Available local services, social networks	Volunteer services, community programs

Support System Assessment

Internal Resources

- Family member availability
- Extended family support
- Friend networks
- Religious community
- Neighborhood connections

External Resources

- Social services
- Community programs
- Religious organizations
- Volunteer services
- Support groups

Identifying Gaps

Common Areas Requiring Support

- 24-hour caregiving coverage
- Respite care needs
- Transportation assistance
- Meal preparation
- Household maintenance

Remember that family resource assessment is ongoing, as needs and available supports may change throughout the hospice journey. Regular reassessment helps ensure continuous appropriate support for both patient and family.

Team Coordination

Effective team coordination ensures seamless delivery of support services while maximizing patient and family outcomes. Clear communication and structured collaboration among team members create a comprehensive care approach.

Core Team Components

Primary Care Team

- Case Manager
- Primary Nurse
- Hospice Aide
- Social Worker
- Chaplain
- Medical Director

Extended Support Team

- Volunteers
- Therapists
- Pharmacist
- Bereavement Counselors
- On-Call Staff

Coordination Strategies

Activity	Frequency	Purpose
IDT Meetings	Weekly	Care plan review and updates
Care Conferences	Every 14 days	Family/team collaboration
Daily Huddles	Each morning	Immediate needs and changes

Activity	Frequency	Purpose
On-Call Reports	Each shift	Continuity of care

Communication Protocols

Essential Information Sharing

- Changes in condition
- New symptoms or concerns
- Family dynamics
- Resource needs
- Care plan updates

Documentation Requirements

- Team communications
- Care coordination efforts
- Service delivery updates
- Follow-up needs
- Outcome measurements

Role Delineation

Clear Definition of Responsibilities

- Primary contact assignments
- Service coordination leads
- Communication channels
- Decision-making authority
- Emergency protocols

Remember that effective team coordination directly impacts the quality of care delivery and family satisfaction with hospice services.

Quality Measures

Coordination Effectiveness

- Response times
- Service integration

- Family Satisfaction
- Care plan adherence
- Team collaboration

Successful team coordination ensures comprehensive care delivery while supporting optimal patient and family outcomes.

Documentation Requirements

Proper documentation of support services ensures regulatory compliance, demonstrates service value, and facilitates effective care coordination. Clear, comprehensive documentation supports quality care delivery while meeting Medicare requirements.

Essential Documentation Elements

Service Delivery Documentation

- Type of service provided
- Duration of service
- Provider identification
- Patient/family response
- Follow-up needs

Support Service Assessment

- Identified needs
- Services offered
- Services accepted/declined
- Effectiveness evaluation
- Plan modifications

Required Timeframes

Documentation Type	When Required	Purpose
Initial Assessment	Within 5 days	Establish baseline needs
Service Updates	Every visit	Track utilization

Documentation Type	When Required	Purpose
Team Communication	Within 24 hours	Ensure coordination
Care Plan Updates	Every 15 days	Monitor effectiveness
Discharge Planning	Ongoing	Ensure continuity

Medicare Requirements

Key Components

- Service necessity
- Appropriate interventions
- Response to services
- Ongoing need
- Cost-effectiveness

Quality Assurance Elements

Documentation Must Be

- Clear and specific
- Timely and complete
- Objective and accurate
- Properly authenticated
- Readily accessible

Remember that thorough documentation supports service continuation, demonstrates value, and ensures regulatory compliance while facilitating team communication.

Best Practices

Documentation Guidelines

- Use approved terminology
- Include all required elements
- Document promptly
- Maintain confidentiality
- Follow organizational policies

Effective documentation of support services ensures continuity of care while supporting regulatory compliance and quality assurance efforts.

Conclusion to Chapter 7: Maximizing Support Services

Maximizing support services requires a thoughtful, comprehensive approach that begins with holistic assessment and extends through careful documentation. Your expertise in identifying needs, coordinating services, and ensuring effective team communication helps create a network of support that enhances the hospice experience for both patients and families.

Remember that each support service you coordinate represents an opportunity to improve the quality of life and provide relief to caregivers. By implementing thorough assessments, effectively utilizing available services, evaluating family resources carefully, maintaining strong team coordination, and documenting appropriately, you help fulfill hospice's promise of comprehensive care.

Your role in maximizing support services demonstrates the essence of hospice care - meeting patients' medical needs and supporting the family's physical, emotional, social, and spiritual needs. This comprehensive approach truly makes a difference in the lives of those we serve.

Conclusion: Achieving Excellence in Hospice Care

Excellence in hospice care represents more than just following protocols and meeting regulations - it embodies our commitment to providing exceptional end-of-life care that honors each patient's journey while supporting their loved ones.

Key Takeaways

The foundation of excellent hospice care rests on several critical elements:

- Early recognition of decline through careful assessment
- Proactive rather than reactive care delivery
- Comprehensive care planning that adapts to changing needs
- Effective medication and symptom management
- Maximizing support services for patients and families
- Clear communication and thorough documentation

Implementation Strategies

Excellence requires consistent application of best practices:

- Systematic visit approaches that ensure comprehensive care
- Regular evaluation of care plan effectiveness
- Proactive identification of needs and potential issues
- Strong team coordination and communication
- Continuous family education and support
- Thorough documentation that supports quality care

Quality Metrics and Outcomes

Success in hospice care is measured through:

- Patient comfort and symptom management
- Family satisfaction and support
- Prevention of crisis situations
- Appropriate utilization of services

- Regulatory compliance
- Team collaboration effectiveness

Call to Action for Excellence

As hospice nurses, we are called to:

- Maintain the highest standards of care
- Continuously enhance our skills and knowledge
- Support and mentor colleagues
- Advocate for patient and family needs
- Contribute to the advancement of hospice care
- Demonstrate compassion in all interactions

Continuing Education Resources

Excellence requires ongoing professional development:

- Professional organization memberships
- Certification opportunities
- Educational conferences
- Online learning platforms
- Peer mentoring programs
- Current research and literature

Remember that excellence in hospice care is not a destination but a continuous journey of growth, learning, and dedication to serving patients and families during one of life's most significant transitions.

Your commitment to excellence makes a profound difference in the lives of those we serve, honoring both the privilege and responsibility of providing end-of-life care.

Appendix A: Assessment Checklists

Initial Visit Assessment Checklist

Patient Assessment

- ☐ Vital signs and current symptoms
- ☐ Level of consciousness
- ☐ Pain assessment
- ☐ Functional status (PPS/KPS)
- ☐ Skin assessment
- ☐ Nutritional status
- ☐ Safety evaluation

Medication Review

- ☐ Current medication list
- ☐ Effectiveness evaluation
- ☐ Side effects assessment
- ☐ Storage conditions
- ☐ Supply status
- ☐ Comfort kit review

Environment Assessment

- ☐ Home safety
- ☐ Equipment needs
- ☐ Fall risks
- ☐ Emergency access
- ☐ Temperature control

Routine Visit Checklist

Assessment Area	Key Elements	Documentation Needed
Physical Status	Vital signs, symptoms, changes	Current findings
Medications	Supply, effectiveness, side effects	Updates and needs
Equipment	Functionality, appropriateness	Maintenance/changes
Support Services	Utilization, effectiveness	Service adjustments
Education	Understanding, compliance	Topics covered

Change in Condition Checklist

Immediate Assessment Needs

- ☐ New symptoms
- ☐ Vital sign changes
- ☐ Mental status changes
- ☐ Pain status
- ☐ Respiratory status
- ☐ Medication effectiveness

Support System Evaluation

- ☐ Caregiver coping
- ☐ Resource needs
- ☐ Education requirements
- ☐ Team communication needs
- ☐ Emergency planning

End-of-Life Checklist

Physical Signs

- ☐ Breathing changes
- ☐ Circulation changes
- ☐ Level of consciousness
- ☐ Pain status
- ☐ Skin changes
- ☐ Output changes

Support Requirements

- ☐ Medication needs
- ☐ Equipment needs
- ☐ Family support
- ☐ Spiritual care
- ☐ Team coordination

Remember that these checklists serve as guides and should be adapted based on individual patient needs and organizational requirements.

Quality Assurance Checklist

Visit Documentation

- ☐ Complete assessment
- ☐ Interventions provided
- ☐ Education delivered
- ☐ Follow-up plans
- ☐ Team communication

These comprehensive checklists help ensure thorough assessments and appropriate care delivery while meeting regulatory requirements.

Appendix B: Documentation Templates

Initial Visit Documentation Template

Patient Demographics

- Name, age, diagnosis
- Location of care
- Primary caregiver
- Emergency contacts
- Advance directives

Assessment Findings

Chief Complaint:

History of Present Illness:

Current Symptoms:

Vital Signs:

Physical Assessment:

Functional Status (PPS/KPS):

Pain Assessment:

Care Planning

Problems Identified:

Goals Established:

Interventions Planned:

Education Provided:

Follow-up Needed:

Routine Visit Template

Section	Content Requirements	Examples
Subjective	Patient/caregiver report	"Caregiver reports increased pain..."
Objective	Clinical findings	"VS: BP 120/80, P 72, R 18..."
Assessment	Clinical interpretation	"Patient showing signs of..."
Plan	Interventions and follow-up	"Will increase visits to 2x/week..."

Change in Condition Template

Situation

    Change Identified:

    Onset:

    Severity:

    Impact on Function:

Background

    Relevant History:

    Recent Changes:

    Current Medications:

    Support Systems:

Assessment

    Clinical Findings:

Contributing Factors:

Risk Assessment:

Family Coping:

Recommendations

Interventions:

Education:

Follow-up Plan:

Team Notifications:

End-of-Life Documentation Template

Status Changes

Physical Changes:

Comfort Level:

Medication Response:

Family Coping:

Interventions

Comfort Measures:

Family Support:

Team Communication:

Resource Utilization:

Remember that these templates serve as guides and should be customized to meet your organization's requirements while ensuring comprehensive patient care documentation.

Quality Documentation Elements

Every Visit Must Include

- Changes since the last visit
- Current assessment findings
- Interventions provided
- Response to care
- Plan updates
- Family Education
- Team communication

These templates support thorough documentation while meeting regulatory requirements and promoting quality care delivery. The book ***Compliance-based, Eligibility Driven Hospice Documentation: Tips for Hospice Nurses*** explores quality compliance-driven documentation in more detail.

Appendix C: Communication Scripts

Initial Visit Introduction

First Contact

"Hello, I'm [Name] from [Hospice Agency]. I'm your hospice nurse, and I'm here to help support you and your family during this time. May I come in and talk with you about how we can best help?"

Setting Expectations

"Let me explain how hospice care works and what you can expect from our team. We're here to ensure comfort and support for both [Patient Name] and your family. Do you have any immediate concerns we should address?"

Discussing Changes in Condition

Decline Recognition

"I've noticed some changes in [Patient Name]'s condition that I'd like to discuss with you. These changes include [specific observations]. This often means [explanation of significance]. What changes have you noticed?"

End-of-Life Approaching

"Based on the changes we're seeing, I want to help prepare you for what might come next. Would it be okay if we talked about what to expect and how we can best support you through this?"

Crisis Prevention

Situation	Script	Follow-up
Pain Management	"If pain increases, first try [intervention]. If that doesn't help within [timeframe], call us at..."	Document understanding
Breathing Changes	"If you notice [specific changes], here's what to do first. Then call us if..."	Verify comfort with plan
Medication Issues	"Before running out of medications, call us when you have a [timeframe] supply left..."	Confirm understanding

Family Education

Medication Teaching

"Let me show you how to give this medication. I'll demonstrate first, then guide you through it. Feel free to ask questions at any point."

Comfort Measures

"There are several ways we can help keep [Patient Name] comfortable. Let's go through each option, and you can tell me what works best for your situation."

Difficult Conversations

Addressing Fears

"Many families worry about [common concern]. Would you like to talk about what concerns you most? We can work together to address these concerns."

Explaining Decline

"When we see these changes, it often means [explanation]. This helps us plan better for [Patient Name]'s care. What questions do you have about these changes?"

Support Service Introduction

Team Member Roles

> "Our team includes several specialists who can help in different ways. For example, our social worker can assist with [specific services], and our chaplain can provide [specific support]. Would you like to learn more about any of these services?"

Remember that these scripts serve as guides and should be adapted to your personal style and the specific needs of each patient and family. The key is maintaining a compassionate, professional tone while ensuring clear communication.

Phone Communication

After-Hours Calls

> "This is [Name], the on-call hospice nurse. I understand you're calling about [concern]. Can you tell me more about what's happening right now?"

Follow-up Calls

> "I'm calling to check on how things are going since our visit yesterday. How has [Patient Name] been doing with [specific concern]?"

These communication scripts help ensure consistent, professional, and compassionate interaction with patients and families while promoting clear understanding and cooperation.

Appendix D: Quick Reference Guides

Common Symptom Management

Symptom	First-Line Interventions	When to Escalate
Pain	PRN oral medication, positioning	Unrelieved after 2 doses
Dyspnea	Position changes, fan, oxygen	Increased distress
Anxiety	Reassurance, calm environment	Increasing agitation
Nausea	Small sips, cool cloths	Unable to take medications
Confusion	Reorientation, familiar faces	New onset, sudden change

Medication Conversion Guide

Opioid Equivalents

- Morphine 30mg oral = 15mg IV/SQ
- Hydromorphone 7.5mg oral = 1.5mg IV/SQ
- Oxycodone 20mg oral = 30mg oral morphine

Vital Sign Parameters

When to Report

- Temperature > 101.5°F
- Systolic BP < 90 or > 180
- Heart rate < 50 or > 120
- Respiratory rate < 8 or > 28
- O2 sat < 88% (if monitoring)

Emergency Kit Guidelines

Contents Check

- Morphine/appropriate opioid
- Anti-anxiety medication
- Anti-nausea medication
- Anti-secretory medication
- Fever reducer

Usage Criteria

- Symptoms matching medication
- Following order parameters
- Documentation requirements
- Replacement process

DME Quick Guide

Common Equipment Needs

- Hospital bed: Unable to transfer safely
- Oxygen: Dyspnea, O2 sat < 88% if the patient is uncomfortable
- Wheelchair: Limited mobility
- Bedside commode: Unable to reach bathroom
- Shower chair: Fall risk

Visit Frequency Guidelines

Status	Suggested Frequency	Indicators
Stable	1-2x/week	Symptoms controlled
Declining	2-3x/week	New symptoms
Imminent	Daily	Active dying
Crisis	Multiple/day	Uncontrolled symptoms

Documentation Essentials

Every Visit Must Include

- Vital signs (as appropriate)
- Pain assessment
- Symptom management
- Medication review
- Supply check
- Family Education
- Follow-up plan

Communication Chain

Urgent Issues

1. On-call nurse
2. Case manager
3. Team manager
4. Medical director

Non-urgent Issues

1. Case manager
2. IDT meeting
3. Team lead

Remember, these quick references are guides and should be used with your organization's policies and procedures.

Medicare Requirements

Visit Documentation Must Show

- Skilled need
- Changes in condition
- Response to interventions
- Plan modifications
- Family Education

References and Resources

What Hospice Nurses should assess every visit at https://compassioncrossing.info/what-hospice-nurses-should-assess-every-visit/

Frequency of Changes in Condition as an Indicator of Approaching Death at https://compassioncrossing.info/velocity-of-changes-in-condition-as-an-indicator-of-approaching-death/

Understanding Functional Decline in the Natural Dying Process at https://compassioncrossing.info/understanding-functional-decline-in-the-natural-dying-process/

Breathing Patterns Before End of Life: Critical Clues for the Last Hours! at https://compassioncrossing.info/breathing-pattern-before-end-of-life-critical-clue-for-the-last-hours/

Significant Signs a Terminally Ill Patient may be Close to Dying at https://compassioncrossing.info/significant-signs-a-terminally-ill-patient-may-be-close-to-dying/

Trigger Words for Hospice Nurses: Assessing End-of-Life in Two Weeks or Less at https://compassioncrossing.info/trigger-words-for-hospice-nurses-assessing-end-of-life-in-two-weeks-or-less/

Understanding Changes in Palliative Performance Scale in the Last Six Months of Life at https://compassioncrossing.info/understanding-changes-in-palliative-performance-scale-in-the-last-six-months-of-life/

Understanding the Patient's Question: When Will I Die? at https://compassioncrossing.info/how-best-to-address-the-most-common-question-in-hospice-when/

Understanding Terminal Illness Progression: Observable Signs and Symptoms at https://compassioncrossing.info/understanding-terminal-illness-progression-observable-signs-and-symptoms/

Understanding Nutrition Changes in Hospice: Nourishing Comfort and Peaceful End-of-Life Journey at https://compassioncrossing.info/understanding-nutrition-changes-in-hospice-nourishing-comfort-and-peaceful-end-of-life-journey/

Sleeping as a Prognostication Tool for the Terminally Ill at https://compassioncrossing.info/sleeping-as-a-prognostication-tool-for-the-terminally-ill/

The Final Journey: Understanding Why the Actively Dying May Linger at https://compassioncrossing.info/the-final-journey-understanding-why-the-actively-dying-may-linger/

Understanding the Common Journey Towards End-of-Life at https://compassioncrossing.info/understanding-the-common-journey-towards-end-of-life/

The Dying Process at the End of Life at https://compassioncrossing.info/the-dying-process-at-the-end-of-life/

The last hours of life at https://compassioncrossing.info/the-last-hours-of-life/

Educational Topics for Hospice Nurses During Admission and Post-Admission Visits at https://compassioncrossing.info/educational-topics-for-hospice-nurses-during-admission-and-post-admission-visits/

Understanding KPS and PPS: Vital Assessment Tools in Palliative and Hospice Care at https://compassioncrossing.info/understanding-kps-and-pps-vital-assessment-tools-in-palliative-and-hospice-care/

Hospice Nursing Visit Frequencies: A Guide for New Hospice Nurses at https://compassioncrossing.info/nursing-visit-frequencies-on-hospice-a-guide-for-new-hospice-nurses/

The Sunset Assessment Scale for Determining Hospice Skilled Nursing Visit Frequencies at https://compassioncrossing.info/the-sunset-assessment-scale-for-determining-hospice-skilled-nursing-visit-frequencies/

How to Talk to Families About End-of-Life: A Guide for Hospice Nurses at https://compassioncrossing.info/how-to-talk-to-families-about-end-of-life-a-guide-for-hospice-nurses/

Understanding the Importance of Quarterly Medication Reconciliation for Terminal Patients at https://compassioncrossing.info/understanding-the-importance-of-quarterly-medication-reconciliation-for-terminal-patients/

Crisis Management at End-of-Life at https://compassioncrossing.info/crisis-management-at-end-of-life/

Hospice Pharmacy Utilization Management Strategies Support Quality Care at https://enclarapharmacia.com/hospice-pharmacy-utilization-management-strategies-support-quality-care

Measuring the Quality of Hospice Care at https://www.ahrq.gov/talkingquality/measures/setting/long-term-care/hospice.html

Creating An Effective Hospice Plan of Care at https://www.cms.gov/files/document/mln9895410-creating-effective-hospice-plan-care.pdf

How Hospice Nurses Build Trust With Patients and Families at https://www.nurse.com/blog/hospice-nurse-builds-trust-nsp/

STEADI - Older Adult Fall Prevention at https://www.cdc.gov/steadi/hcp/clinical-resources/index.html

Compliance-based, Eligibility Driven Hospice Documentation: Tips for Hospice Nurses at https://amzn.to/4fb9L9k

Whispers of Time: Understanding the End-of-Life Timeline at https://amzn.to/3SnfeA4

Mastering Hospice Eligibility: An Essential Guide for RNs and Clinical Managers at https://amzn.to/47tA8UE

Mastering Hospice Recertifications: A Comprehensive Guide for Nurses at https://amzn.to/3z1ls2i

Conversations at the End: Guiding Families Through Final Days at https://amzn.to/3ziXUpy

Mastering the Hospice Item Set: A Comprehensive Guide for Nurses and Managers at https://amzn.to/3XloiHs

Care Plans for Hospice Patients: A Comprehensive Guide at https://amzn.to/3XxLJNW

Mindful Minutes: Time Management Secrets for Hospice Nursing Excellence at https://amzn.to/4eGfLFY

Medication Reconciliation in Hospice Care: Maximizing Quality of Life at https://amzn.to/3Y6MyyF

HOPE in Practice: Implementing Patient-Centered Outcomes in Hospice Care at https://amzn.to/3YfhGMB

Author Bio

Peter Abraham, BSN, RN is an experienced nurse dedicated to supporting nurses, caregivers, families, and patients in their learning, growth, and well-being journey. Peter's nursing path encompasses practical experience as a cardiac telemetry nurse in a bustling cardiology unit at a Magnet-awarded teaching hospital. Additionally, Peter has fulfilled the role of a second-shift RN supervisor, overseeing an entire building in an SNF/LTC (Skilled Nursing Facility/Long-Term Care) setting with 151 residents. Remarkably, during the initial wave of COVID-19, the facility achieved an impressive close-to-100% recovery rate before operation warp speed was complete.

Furthermore, Peter's nursing career extends to rural home hospice care. As a visiting hospice registered nurse case manager, he offers compassionate care to patients in various settings, including private homes, personal care homes, assisted living facilities, skilled nursing facilities, and hospitals.

Moreover, Peter's desire to help others extends beyond his physical presence. At CompassionCrossing.Info, he writes articles to empower caregivers, family members, and fellow nurses in end-of-life care. Peter's drive to help others, which flows from his love of Christ Jesus, is a source of support and encouragement for all he reaches.

Other books by Peter Abraham include the following:

Empowering Excellence in Hospice: A Nurse's Toolkit for Best Practices series:

>Compliance-based, Eligibility Driven Hospice Documentation: Tips for Hospice Nurses
>Whispers of Time: Understanding the End-of-Life Timeline
>Mastering Hospice Eligibility: An Essential Guide for RNs and Clinical Managers
>Mastering Recertifications: A Comprehensive Guide for Nurses
>Conversations at the End: Guiding Families Through Final Days
>Mastering the Hospice Item Set: A Comprehensive Guide for Nurses and Managers
>Care Plans for Hospice Patients: A Comprehensive Guide
>Mindful Minutes: Time Management Secrets for Hospice Nursing Excellence
>Medication Reconciliation in Hospice Care: Maximizing Quality of Life
>HOPE in Practice: Implementing Patient-Centered Outcomes in Hospice Care
>The Complete Hospice Visit: A Nurse's Guide to Excellence

Compassionate Caregiving series:

>Daily Hospice Care Planner: Organize, Communicate, and Provide Consistent Care
>Dignity in Dying: A Thoughtful Approach to Voluntary Stopping Eating and Drinking
>Palliative Sedation: A Compassionate Approach
>Hospice Medication Handbook: A Caregiver's Guide to Comfort Medications
>Nourishing Hope: A Caregiver's Guide to End-of-Life Nutrition
>Validation and Compassion: A Guide to Connecting with Terminally Ill Loved Ones
>Palliative Care vs Hospice Care: Making Informed Decisions
>Understanding Your Rights in Hospice Care: A Guide for Patients and Families
>
>When It's Time for Hospice: A Compassionate Guide for Families and Caregivers
>The Caregiver's Lifeline: Self-Care in End-of-Life Care

Dementia Caregivers Essentials series:

Dementia Caregiver Essentials (all ten books below in one)

Anger Management in Dementia
CPAP and Oxygen for Dementia
Diabetes Care for Dementia
Hallucination Management for Dementia
Infection Awareness in Dementia
Medication Compliance for Dementia
Music Therapy for Dementia
Nutrition for Dementia
Placement for Dementia
Sundowning Management for Dementia

Holistic Nurse: Skills for Excellence series

Compassionate Care in Conflict: A Nurse's Guide to Managing Combative Patients
Dementia Staging Mastery: A Nurse's Guide to Dementia Assessment
The Nurse's Guide to Motivational Interviewing: Empowering Patients to Make Lasting Health Changes

The above books can be found on Amazon at https://amzn.to/3YFBYQ0

Connect with Peter On:

Website: https://compassioncrossing.info/

www.ingramcontent.com/pod-product-compliance
Lightning Source LLC
Chambersburg PA
CBHW071059240526
45471CB00016B/2165